Med. N67/17
7/93

CHARLES FREARS COLLEGE
C011598

WITHDRAWN
DE MONTFORT UNIVERSITY
LIBRARY

HARLES FREARS COLLEGE OF
NURSING AND MIDWIFERY
EARNING RESOURCES CENTRE

TANDARDIZED NURSING CARE PLANS FOR EMERGENCY DEPARTMENTS

te sh... below

STANDARDIZED NURSING CARE PLANS FOR EMERGENCY DEPARTMENTS

PAMELA BOURG, R.N., M.S., C.E.N.

Assistant Director of Nursing, Emergency Medical Services and Outpatient Department, Denver General Hospital; Assistant Clinical Professor, University of Colorado Health Sciences Center, Denver, Colorado

CAROLEE SHERER, R.N., M.S., C.E.N.

Nursing Unit Administrator, Emergency Department, University Hospital, University of Colorado Health Sciences Center, Denver, Colorado

PETER ROSEN, M.D.

Director, Emergency Medical Services, Denver General Hospital; Professor, Emergency Medicine, Surgery Department, University of Colorado Health Sciences Center, Denver, Colorado

Illustrated

THE C. V. MOSBY COMPANY

ST. LOUIS • WASHINGTON, D.C. • TORONTO 1986

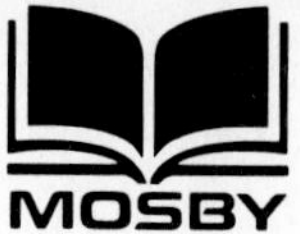

A TRADITION OF PUBLISHING EXCELLENCE

Editor: Barbara Ellen Norwitz
Developmental editor: Sally Adkisson
Editing/Production: Helen C. Hudlin
Design: Kay M. Kram

DE MONTFORT UNIVERSITY LIBRARY
CLASS: 616.025 BOU
Re-classified to Dewey in 2010

WB 105 BOU

C011598

Copyright © 1986 by The C.V. Mosby Company

All rights reserved. No part of this publication may be reproduced, stored in a retrieval system, or transmitted, in any form or by any means, electronic, mechanical, photocopying, recording, or otherwise, without prior written permission from the publisher.

Printed in the United States of America

The C.V. Mosby Company
11830 Westline Industrial Drive, St. Louis, Missouri 63146

Library of Congress Cataloging-in-Publication Data

Standardized nursing care plans for emergency departments.

Bibliography: p.
Includes index.
1. Emergency nursing—Planning. 2. Nursing care plans. I. Bourg, Pamela W. II. Sherer, Carolee. III. Rosen, Peter, 1935-
RT120.E4S73 1986 610.73'61 86-5407
ISBN 0-8016-1257-8

VT/VH/VH 9 8 7 6 5 4 3 2 01/A/091

CONTRIBUTORS

TERRY ANDERSON, R.N., C.E.N.*

Clinical Nurse,
Longmont Medical Center,
Lafayette, Colorado

MARTI BOATRIGHT, R.N., M.S.*

Station Nurse Manager,
Park Hill Health Station,
Department of Health and Hospitals,
City of Denver,
Denver, Colorado

PAMELA BOURG, R.N., M.S., C.E.N.

Assistant Director of Nursing,
Emergency Medical Services and Outpatient Department,
Denver General Hospital;
Assistant Clinical Professor,
University of Colorado Health Sciences Center,
Denver, Colorado

MARILYN BOURN, R.N., B.S.N., C.E.N.*

Manager,
Community Medical Center,
Lafayette, Colorado

ANN BURRIS, R.N.

Former Clinical Nurse,
Denver General Hospital,
Denver, Colorado

STEPHEN CANTRILL, M.D.

Attending Physician,
Emergency Medical Services,
Denver General Hospital,
Denver, Colorado

*Former Clinical Nurse, Denver General Hospital, Denver, Colorado.

GEORGIA CAVEN, R.N., B.S., C.C.R.N., C.E.N.
Clinical Nurse,
Emergency Department,
Denver General Hospital,
Denver, Colorado

ANN CHAMBERS, R.N., B.S.*
Head Nurse,
Hartford Regional Center,
Hartford, Connecticut

CYNTHIA DEPIES, R.N., B.S.*
Clinical Nurse,
Recovery Room,
Denver General Hospital,
Denver, Colorado

NANCY FISTLER, R.N., B.S.*
Clinical Nurse,
Intensive Care,
Denver Presbyterian Hospital,
Denver, Colorado

DENISE GORNICK, R.N.
Former Clinical Nurse,
Denver General Hospital,
Denver, Colorado

DONNA HELGREN, R.N., C.E.N.
Clinical Nurse,
Emergency Department,
Denver General Hospital,
Denver, Colorado

DEBORAH JANTZEN, R.N.*
Flight Nurse,
St. Anthony's Hospital Systems,
Denver, Colorado

ROBERT JORDAN, M.D.
Director, Division of Emergency Medicine,
University of Mississippi;
Associate Professor of Medicine,
University of Mississippi School of Medicine,
Jackson, Mississippi

*Former Clinical Nurse, Denver General Hospital, Denver, Colorado.

DEBORAH KLAISLE, R.N., M.D.*

Intern,
University of Colorado Health Sciences Center,
Denver, Colorado

DOROTHEA LOUX, R.N.*

Clinical Nurse,
Emergency Department,
San Francisco General,
San Francisco, California

MICHELLE MALMGREN, R.N., B.S.N., C.E.N.

Clinical Nurse,
Denver General Hospital,
Denver, Colorado

VINCENT MARKOVCHICK, M.D.

Assistant Director of Emergency Medicine,
Emergency Medical Services,
Denver General Hospital,
Denver, Colorado

DONNA MARSHALL, R.N., C.E.N.*

Administrative Office,
Cost Containment Division,
Colorado Medicaid Bureau,
Denver, Colorado

JOHN MARX, M.D.

Attending Physician,
Emergency Medical Services,
Denver General Hospital,
Denver, Colorado

CHRIS MAY, R.N., M.S.N., C.E.N.*

Education Coordinator,
Ambulatory Services,
Kettering Medical Center,
Kettering, Ohio

ALICE McLARNON, R.N., C.E.N.

Assistant Head Nurse,
Emergency Department,
Denver General Hospital,
Denver, Colorado

*Former Clinical Nurse, Denver General Hospital, Denver, Colorado.

JUDY McLEAN, R.N.
Clinical Nurse,
Emergency Department,
Denver General Hospital,
Denver, Colorado

ELIZABETH O'FLAHERTY, R.N., B.S.N.
Assistant Nursing Unit Administrator,
Emergency Department,
University Hospital,
University of Colorado Health Sciences Center,
Denver, Colorado

KATHY OMAN, R.N., B.S.N.
Clinical Nurse,
Emergency Department,
Denver General Hospital,
Denver, Colorado

PETER PONS, M.D.
Associate Director of Emergency Department,
University Hospital; Assistant Clinical Professor,
University of Colorado Health Sciences Center,
Denver, Colorado

MARY SCHNEIDER, R.N., B.S.N.
Clinical Nurse,
Emergency Department,
Denver General Hospital,
Denver, Colorado

DOROTHY SCHULTE, R.N., B.S.N., C.E.N.
Staff Nurse,
Rocky Mountain Poison Center,
Denver, Colorado

CAROLEE SHERER, R.N., M.S., C.E.N.*
Nursing Unit Administrator,
Emergency Department,
University Hospital,
University of Colorado Health Sciences Center,
Denver, Colorado

FRED SINGER, R.N., B.S.N.
Clinical Nurse,
Emergency Department,
Denver General Hospital,
Denver, Colorado

*Former Clinical Nurse, Denver General Hospital, Denver, Colorado.

JULIE SMITH, R.N., B.S.N., C.E.N.

Assistant Head Nurse,
Emergency Department,
Denver General Hospital,
Denver, Colorado

MARY LOU STEELE, R.N., C.E.N.*

Nursing Supervisor,
After Hours Clinic,
Kaiser Permanente,
Denver, Colorado

KAREN WHITE, R.N.*

Clinical Nurse,
Emergency Department,
North Shore University Hospital,
Manhasset, New York

*Former Clinical Nurse, Denver General Hospital, Denver, Colorado.

ɔ the nurses, clerks, and orderlies in the Emergency Department at
enver General Hospital, who daily strive for excellence in emergency care

ɔ my personal and professional family
ne nurses, physicians, and paramedics who have fostered my knowledge
nd interest in emergency care, and especially to Mom, Dad, and Jolene,
whom I owe my beginnings, my education, and my ambition.

CJS

FOREWORD

As I think back on my nursing career—which now spans two decades—when the term "care plans" is mentioned, my mind automatically skips back to my student nurse days. How well I can remember the long nights and early mornings spent writing care plans in preparation for the next day's clinical practice and patient care activities. I vividly remember agonizing over the details of care, hoping I didn't leave anything out for fear my instructor would think I wouldn't be a good nurse.

I naively assumed that, once nursing school was through, the agony of preparing care plans would also end. Much to my disgruntled surprise, I learned that care plans were an essential part of daily professional practice and not simply a nursing school activity. As the years went by, I learned to appreciate and depend on care plans, realizing that they were truly beneficial in evaluating and planning care of patients.

In emergency nursing, because of the relative urgency of problems and the chief complaints with which patients present, there is usually *not* time to sit and write *detailed* care plans. Subjective and objective observations must be made rapidly, assessments formulated just as rapidly, and plans implemented in very short periods of time. Add to that the variety of chief complaints one will deal with on a daily basis and emergency nursing becomes an incredible challenge. It is my opinion that this is a major part of the intrigue and attractiveness of emergency nursing—split-second decision-making and interventions based on rapid data gathering.

Perhaps many of us (practicing emergency nurses) have developed some protocols, standing orders, or care plans for patients that we use in our daily practice. Kudos and thanks to Pam Bourg, Carolee Sherer, and Peter Rosen, the authors of this text, for developing *detailed* care plans (based on chief complaints) that are comprehensive and educational as well as for providing us with a condensed but thorough review of the most common chief complaints patients present with in the emergency care setting. They have saved many of us hours, days, weeks, and months of library research and the writing time on a project we have "been meaning to do but just haven't gotten around to yet."

A brief word of caution when using standardized care plans—keep a open mind and allow for variances. Chief complaints and nursing diagnoses ca change rapidly. Care plans are meant as *guidelines* only. Avoid a totally "coo book" approach to emergency nursing. Use these care plans wisely, keep all your senses astute to changes, and your mind open to a rapid change of plans required.

I wish you all much professional satisfaction in your daily practice successes with your resuscitations, and excitement about being emergenc nurses.

Susan Budassi Sheehy, R.N., M.S.N., C.E.N

Assistant Director, Trauma Service
St. Joseph Hospital and Health Care Center
Tacoma, Washington and
Associate Professor of Clinical Nursing
Department of Physiological Nursing
University of Washington
Seattle, Washington

PREFACE

1983 the Emergency Department Nurses Association (now known as ENA) ublished *Standards of emergency nursing practice.** These standards stress e importance of standardizing emergency nursing care and provide guide- nes for the development of specific standards. The standardized care plans in is book evolved out of a need for the nurses at Denver General Hospital to rovide consistent care to patients. These care plans also serve as an instruc- onal guide to orient nurses to what knowledge they must acquire in order to fely care for patients. These care plans can be used as a guide for emergency ursing practice. They are designed to assist nurses in their approach to atients and in dealing with common emergency problems in an organized anner.

Typically the emergency nurse has only a symptom or complaint with hich to be concerned when initiating nursing care. With this in mind, this mergency nursing manual revolves around the complaints of patients as they nter the emergency care system and indicates the proper nursing responses these complaints. The nurse can use this manual to obtain the necessary formation to readily identify what further data needs to be collected and en how to plan and implement emergency nursing care.

It is common practice today for triage systems in most emergency settings separate the trauma-related emergencies from nontrauma emergencies. art I of this book includes the nontrauma care plans and Part II the trauma are plans. The care plans within each part are presented in alphabetical order y symptom; they contain the following components:

Implications for Action: Provides an overview of the importance of the condition. In certain circumstances symptoms are described that require immediate intervention by the nurse.

Assessment: Facilitates the collection of subjective and objective data by the nurse.

Standards of emergency nursing practice, St. Louis, 1983, The C.V. Mosby Company.

Diagnoses/Analysis: Lists possible nursing diagnoses related to th health problem.

Planning: Lists priorities of care and includes a differential assessme and management section that describes potential medical diagnose specific clinical assessment parameters, and specific nursing actio to be taken.

Implementation: Spells out primary and secondary nursing actions to b taken, including medications and dosages.

Evaluation: Details patient outcome criteria to be used in evaluati nursing care and to direct the nurse to reevaluate the interventions patient outcomes are not reached.

Disposition: Outlines admission criteria and instructions for discharg

Most of the information is presented in an outline format so that it may b quickly and easily retrieved.

The six-step nursing process, including nursing diagnosis, serves as th framework for the care plans. The use of the nursing diagnosis has been ide tified as a standard of practice by the Emergency Nurses Association (ENA) i its *Standards of emergency nursing practice.* Such use enables the nurse t identify patient care needs, aids in establishing priorities for care, and facil tates the selection of appropriate nursing interventions. Thus the nursing dia nosis guides the planning and implementation of specific nursing therapies an facilitates identification of patient outcomes necessary for the evaluation nursing care.

In using nursing diagnosis in the emergency department, the emergenc nurse must be aware of the nurse practice act of his/her individual state. No all states recognize the term "nursing diagnosis." The law is concerned wit the treatment after the diagnosis is made. If the appropriate diagnosis is mad but inappropriate care is given, legal ramifications are possible. On the othe hand, if the wrong diagnosis is made but correct care is given, the law is no concerned if the breach of duty has not led to harm.*

We wish to acknowledge the following people who made this book reality:

Judy-Jo Wells-Mackie, R.N., M.S., former Clinical Specialist, Emergency Department, Denver General Hospital, who shared the dream of standardized care plans for emergency departments.

*Fortin, J.D., and Rabinow, J.: Legal implications of nursing diagnosis, Nurs. Clin. North Am. **14**:553, 1979.

Linda Topping, Dianne Perez, Erin Gallagher, and **Angie Valdez,** who labored over the many drafts of these standards.

and

Billie Klaus, R.N., M.S., Associate Director of Nursing of Ambulatory Services, Denver General Hospital, who provided encouragement and support for this endeavor.

Pamela Bourg
Carolee Sherer
Peter Rosen

HOW TO USE THIS BOOK

ese standardized care plans indicate broad-based care for the most common nergency problems; they should serve as guides for planning individualized re. In order to gain maximum use of these care plans, the steps below should followed:

1. Identify the symptom or the major injury of the patient and locate the appropriate care plan.
2. Use the "Implications for Action" section to identify specific problems that require immediate attention.
3. Collect the assessment data as outlined in initial observation, subjective, and objective sections.
4. Select the appropriate nursing diagnoses for the individual patient from the list of possibilities.
5. Plan for the priorities of care. The differential section outlines the clinical medical problems that encompass the dependent and interdependent dimension of nursing. The nursing responsibilities are clearly outlined according to specific etiology.
6. Proceed to the "Implementation" section, which identifies specific interventions for the symptoms or injuries. Choose the appropriate interventions based on nursing diagnoses and clinical medical problems. (Not all interventions are for every patient.) The secondary interventions are those actions that can wait until primary interventions are carried out and until the patient is stabilized.
7. Check the patient outcomes. If they are not reached, reevaluate the interventions and change the plan of care accordingly. The patient outcomes can also be used retrospectively to audit the charts and to determine the effectiveness of the nursing care.
8. Document the assessment data, the interventions, and the patient's response.

9. Check the admission criteria to determine if the patient's conditi requires inpatient hospital care.
10. Refer to the discharge instructions and convey the necessary speci information to the patient. Also refer to the discharge instructi sheets that are provided in Appendix E.

CONTENTS

PART ONE

NONTRAUMA CARE PLANS

CHAPTER 1

ABDOMINAL PAIN

MPLICATIONS FOR ACTION

onditions causing abdominal pain may vary from relatively benign entities to n acute abdominal condition requiring surgery. The highest priority is hemo-ynamic stabilization followed by careful assessment to isolate the cause of ain. Patients may be discharged without a definitive source of the pain having een identified. In these cases, however, thorough home care instructions and ssurance of a disposition that includes early reobservation are indicated. The ollowing protocol outlines the priorities for care of the patient with abdomi-al pain.

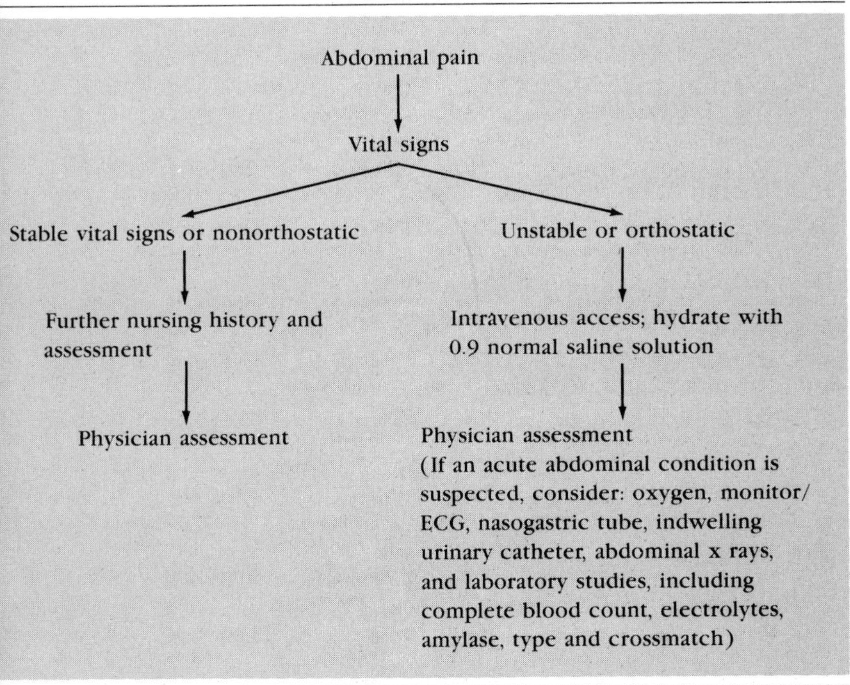

ASSESSMENT

I. Initial observation
   A. Body position and facial expression indicative of pain
   B. Skin color
II. Subjective assessment
   A. Characteristics of pain
      1. Time and nature of onset
      2. Type: sharp, dull, crampy, pressure
      3. Intensity and duration: constant or intermittent
      4. Location and radiation of pain
      5. Aggravating or alleviating factors
      6. Attempted remedies such as antacids
   B. Associated symptoms
      1. Nausea or vomiting, hematemesis, and the relationship of thes symptoms to the onset of pain
      2. Constipation, ostipation, or diarrhea; melena
      3. Belching or flatulence
      4. Urinary frequency, dysuria, or observed hematuria
      5. Fever or chills
      6. Anorexia or weight loss
   C. Gynecological history
      1. Last menstrual period
         a) Date
         b) Normal or abnormal flow
      2. Possibility of pregnancy
         a) Sexually active
         b) Contraception used
         c) Gravity and parity
      3. Vaginal discharge or bleeding
      4. Pain with intercourse
   D. Past medical history
      1. Prior or concurrent illnesses or abdominal surgery
      2. Alcohol or drug abuse
   E. Current medications: especially those, such as aspirin or antiinflamm tory agents, causing gastric side effects
   F. Personal psychosocial stresses

II. Objective assessment
  A. Vital signs
    1. Obtain rectal temperature if patient is unable to cooperate for oral route
    2. Determine orthostatic vital signs if vomiting, diarrhea, or distention is present unless patient is hypotensive when supine
  B. Inspection
    1. Skin color
    2. Scars
    3. Visible masses
    4. Distention
  C. Auscultation
    1. Performed before palpation
    2. Presence and frequency or absence of bowel sounds
    3. Bruits
  D. Palpation
    1. Begun a quadrant away from painful site
    2. Direct or referred pain to palpation
    3. Abdomen soft or firm; guarding: voluntary or involuntary
    4. Masses or organomegaly
    5. Rebound tenderness

POSSIBLE NURSING DIAGNOSES/ANALYSIS

I. Anxiety
II. Bowel elimination, alteration in: constipation, diarrhea
III. Cardiac output, alteration in: decreased
IV. Comfort, alteration in: pain
V. Fluid volume deficit, potential
VI. Knowledge deficit (regarding present illness)
VII. Tissue perfusion, alteration in: cerebral, cardiopulmonary, gastrointestinal, peripheral
VIII. Urinary elimination, alteration in patterns

PLANNING

I. Priorities for care
  A. Hemodynamic management
  B. Isolating cause of abdominal pain
I. Differential management

Condition	Clinical Assessment	Management
GASTROINTESTINAL DISORDERS		
Gastroenteritis	Viral illness resulting in nausea, vomiting, diarrhea, with progression to crampy abdominal pain; may involve fever, chills, muscular aches	Initiate IV hydration if patient is orthostatic; give clear liquid diet and antiemetics; obtain electrolytes and glucose if vomiting or diarrhea is prolonge
Ulcer Disease	Peptic ulcer associated with epigastric pain or with food or hunger; nausea and vomiting; perforation causes peritonitis: acute onset of severe, sharp abdominal pain, rigid abdominal guarding, peristalsis present or absent, hypovolemia	Give antacids, cimetedine; consider bleeding ulcer and obtain hematocrit (re fer to Chapter 11, Care Plan for Gastrointestinal Bleeding); initiate IV hydration; take abdominal x ray to detect free air if perforated; insert nasogastric tube; type and crossmatch; may require surgical intervention
Intestinal Obstruction	Caused by inflammation, adhesions, stricture defect, carcinoma, volvulus, intussusception, neurogenic disturbance, hernia, gallstones; gradual onset of increasingly severe pain; nausea and vomiting, possibly with fecal smell; hyperperistalsis occurs early with diminished bowel sounds as obstruction progresses; constipation or obstipation, often patient has previous history of abdominal surgery; distended abdomen	Initiate IV hydration; obtain complete blood count an electrolytes; insert nasogastric tube and take abdominal x ray; complet obstruction requires surgical intervention
Appendicitis	Gradual onset of diffuse periumbilical pain localizing to right lower quadrant; progression to nausea, vomiting, anorexia, fever; patient most comfortable with knees flexed; elevated white blood count	Obtain IV access, complete blood count, abdominal x ray; may require surgic intervention; repeat whit blood count and hydrate diagnosis is not definitive

›ndition	Clinical Assessment	Management
›od Poisoning	Onset 1-24 hours after ingestion, depending on type of toxin—sudden abdominal pain, cramping, nausea, vomiting, diarrhea	Initiate IV hydration; give antiemetics; condition is usually self-limiting; report to local health department
;SOCIATED ORGAN SYSTEM DISORDERS		
ıolecystitis	Sudden onset of epigastric or right upper quadrant pain that may radiate to right shoulder (pain may increase following fatty food intake), nausea, vomiting, and fever	Initiate IV hydration; insert nasogastric tube; give analgesia; surgery may be required to remove gallstones
ıncreatitis	Gradual onset of left upper quadrant pain that may radiate to shoulder, patient may have nausea and vomiting; abdomen tender to palpation with hypoactive bowel sound; frequently associated with alcohol intake	Confirmed with elevated amylase level; insert nasogastric tube and initiate IV hydration; many narcotics may cause spasm of sphincter of Oddi; meperidine is preferred drug
ıptured Spleen	May occur in any disease causing splenomegaly; hematoma may form before rupture into peritoneal cavity; sudden onset of left quadrant pain with radiation to left shoulder because of diaphragmatic irritation (Kehr's sign); hypotension; tachycardia	Initiate IV hydration; use pneumatic antishock trousers; obtain initial hematocrit, complete blood count, type and crossmatch whole blood; surgical intervention may be required
ASCULAR DISORDERS		
ıscular Occlusion	Ischemic bowel results in gradual onset of abdominal pain, nausea, and vomiting; infarcted bowel occurs within 60 minutes of occlusion; sudden abdominal pain and large blood loss into bowel causes hypotension, tachycardia, abdominal distention	Initiate IV hydration; obtain complete blood count, type and crossmatch; obtain electrolytes; surgical intervention may be required

Condition	Clinical Assessment	Management
Abdominal Aortic Aneurysm	Constant, severe midline back pain, often described as tearing sensation, radiating to back or lower quadrants; palpable pulsating mass; dissection may occur, resulting in tachycardia, hypotension, diaphoresis, and pallor with rapid exsanguination	Obtain hematocrit and initiate IV hydration; use pneumatic antishock trousers; type and crossmatch whole blood; do complete blood count; surgical intervention ma be required
Cardiac-Related Disease	Cardiac pain may be referred to upper abdominal area	(Refer to Chapter 4, Care Plan for Chest Pain)
GYNECOLOGICAL AND GENITOURINARY DISORDERS		
Ectopic Pregnancy	Mild to acute abdominal pain, often localized; patient may have pain radiating to shoulder, vaginal bleeding, often hypotension and tachycardia; late menstrual period or abnormal previous period	Obtain IV access, hematoc type and crossmatch whole blood; confirm wi culdocentesis (refer to Chapter 28, Care Plan fo Vaginal Bleeding and to appendix A for culdocen tesis procedure); surgica intervention may be required
Ovarian Cyst	Onset of pain; similar to signs of ectopic pregnancy; pain usually localized until cyst ruptures; patient may have peritoneal signs and vaginal spotting	Differentiate from ectopic pregnancy; hematocrit le than 15% from culdocen tesis indicates ruptured ovarian cyst; treatment consists primarily of rest
Urinary Tract Infection	Gradual onset of low abdominal and flank pain; dysuria, frequency, urgency, voiding small amounts; patient may have fever and chills	(Refer to Chapter 7, Care Plan for Dysuria); obtain urinalysis
Pelvic Inflammatory Disease	Severe lower abdominal pain, purulent vaginal discharge, fever and chills; infecting organism usually gonococcal	Perform cervical culture; give antibiotics; obtain complete blood count if patient is febrile; positiv cultures required for sex ally transmitted diseases must be reported to loca health department

ondition	Clinical Assessment	Management
enal Colic	Sudden onset of severe, sharp flank pain; may radiate to groin; patient may have total relief between bouts of pain; nausea and vomiting often due to pain; pallor, diaphoresis, tachycardia, restlessness, dysuria	Initiate IV hydration; hemetest urine and strain for stones; perform intravenous pyelogram; give analgesia
esticular Torsion	Torsion of cord results in venous obstruction, venous and arterial thrombosis, and testicular necrosis; sudden pain and edema; erythema of scrotum	Obtain IV access, pain management; surgical intervention may be required
ULMONARY DISORDERS		
	Pain resulting from pneumonia or pulmonary embolus may be referred to abdomen	(Refer to Chapter 22, Care Plan for Respiratory Distress)

MPLEMENTATION

. Primary intervention
   A. Obtain intravenous access for hydration of any patient exhibiting
      1. Hypotension
      2. Orthostasis
      3. Severe distress
   B. Give lactated Ringer's or normal saline (NS) solution rapidly until hypotension or orthostasis resolved
   C. Use slower rates for elderly to avoid fluid overload; observe for tachycardia, shortness of breath, rales
   D. Patient should remain NPO until etiology is identified
   E. Obtain laboratory data and x rays as appropriate according to differential management section

F. Pelvic examination should be done of women with lower abdomin pain
   1. Instruct patient to empty bladder and rectum before examinati and completely undress (privacy should be provided)
   2. Assemble equipment
      a) Speculum
      b) Culture media and slides
      c) Cotton-tipped applicators
      d) Lubricant
      e) Gloves
   3. Assist physician and offer support to patient during examination
   4. Culdocentesis may be required
      a) Diagnostic aid for hemoperitoneum, indicated when ectop pregnancy is suspected
      b) Assemble equipment
         (1) See above
         (2) Local anesthetic
         (3) Spinal needle
         (4) Culdocentesis tray (refer to appendix A)
         (5) Blood tube
      c) Position patient in lithotomy position for pooling
      d) Physician performs aspiration from cul-de-sac
         (1) Positive tap produces nonclotting blood with hematoc less than 15%; venous or arterial blood will clot
         (2) Negative tap—defined by clear serous fluid—does not ru out ectopic pregnancy, which may be unruptured
         (3) Dry tap is nondiagnostic
      e) Evaluation may be required by consulting services such as ge eral surgery or gynecology

II. Secondary intervention
   A. Obtain serial vital signs and assessment of pain
   B. Institute comfort measures; pain medication usually not given un etiology known
   C. Explain to patient and family the progress of evaluation

EVALUATION

I. Patient outcomes/criteria
   A. Vital signs within normal limits
   B. Resolution of orthostasis
   C. Decrease in nausea and vomiting

D. Ability to tolerate oral fluids, if allowed
E. Diminished pain

II. Document initial assessment data, emergency department intervention, and patient's response to treatment

II. If previous patient outcomes are not reached, the emergency nurse should reevaluate the interventions and change the plan of care accordingly

DISPOSITION

I. Admission criteria
   A. Conditions requiring surgical intervention as identified in differential management section
   B. Patients who require a nasogastric tube or who remain NPO because of bowel obstruction, perforated ulcer, or pancreatitis
   C. Patients who are unable to tolerate oral fluids

I. Discharge guidelines
   A. Explain diet instructions, which usually involve giving clear liquids and slowly progressing to solids
   B. Give discharge instructions for (refer to appendix E)
      1. Nausea and vomiting
      2. Urinary tract infection
      3. Pelvic inflammatory disease
   C. Determine follow-up arrangements for gastrointestinal series or ultrasound if appropriate
   D. Dispense medications
   E. Give patient instructions to return if symptoms recur or worsen
   F. Refer to discharge instructions for Abdominal Pain, Vomiting and Diarrhea, Dilation and Curettage, and Urinary Tract Infections in appendix E

CHAPTER 2

ALCOHOL INTOXICATION

IMPLICATIONS FOR ACTION

Assessing the acutely intoxicated patient can prove to be a trying experienc Although reliability of the patient's history may be questionable, presentin complaints cannot be ignored. Protecting the patient from injury is vital sinc normal protective reflexes are lost. Reevaluation is indicated to ensure th patient is becoming more oriented and is exhibiting appropriate behavior. A this occurs, unsuspected disease or injury may become manifest.

Various causes of altered mental status (as outlined in Chapter 27, Ca Plan for the Unresponsive Patient) must be considered. This plan is designed t alert the nurse to special concerns regarding the intoxicated patient an should be used in conjunction with other applicable care plans.

ASSESSMENT

I. Initial observation
   A. Level of consciousness
   B. Respiratory effort
   C. Ataxic gait
II. Subjective assessment
   A. Patient's reason for requesting care
      1. May be unrelated to alcohol, such as chest pain or skeletal pain
      2. Requires appropriate assessment
   B. History should be obtained from a reliable witness such as a famil member or a paramedic
   C. Past medical history
      1. Medications, allergies
      2. Antabuse therapy
      3. Possibility of seizures, trauma, poisoning
   D. Type of alcohol consumed if known; beware of unsuspected isopropy or methanol ingestions
   E. Acute or chronic alcohol intake

I. Objective assessment
  A. Vital signs
    1. Temperature
    2. Orthostatic vital signs if
      a) Patient gives history of fluid loss such as vomiting or diarrhea
      b) Patient is tachycardic
    3. Respiratory status may be diminished with high levels of alcohol
  B. Mental status
    1. Orientation
    2. Impaired thought process or judgment
    3. Type of stimuli necessary for arousal: verbal, touch, painful
    4. Behavior range: from decreased level of consciousness to agitation and combativeness; (BE CAREFUL, alcoholics can harm others as well as themselves)
    5. Slurred speech
  C. Obvious trauma such as lacerations or abrasions
  D. Appearance
    1. Incontinence
    2. Emesis on clothes or body
    3. Nutritional status
  E. Document "patient ataxic with slurred speech" or "odor of alcohol on breath" or "patient admits to alcohol ingestion" rather than claiming "patient is intoxicated"

POSSIBLE NURSING DIAGNOSES/ANALYSIS

I. Airway clearance, ineffective
II. Breathing pattern, ineffective
III. Communication, impaired: verbal
IV. Coping, ineffective individual and family: compromised
V. Fluid volume deficit, actual and potential
VI. Health maintenance, alteration in
VII. Injury: potential for
VIII. Knowledge deficit (effects of alcohol)
IX. Noncompliance
X. Nutrition, alteration in: less than body requirements
XI. Self-concept, disturbance in: body image, self-esteem, role performance, personal identity
XII. Sensory-perceptual alteration: visual
XIII. Social isolation
XIV. Thought processes, alteration in
XV. Violence, potential for: self-directed or directed at others

PLANNING

I. Priorities for care
   A. Protection of airway
   B. Assessment of complaints or injuries
   C. Protection from further injury
   D. Reevaluation when patient is sober

II. Differential management

Condition	Clinical Assessment	Management
ALCOHOL INTOXICATION		
Ethanol	Progression of symptoms: diminished fine motor control, altered sensation, impaired coordination and judgment, delayed reaction time, ataxia, uninhibited behavior, lethargy, coma, respiratory depression	Protect airway; allow patient to sober and then re-evaluate
Methanol and Ethylene Glycol	Epigastric pain, vomiting; results in metabolic acidosis; complications related to toxins of metabolism; methanol ingestion will cause blindness if unrecognized and untreated	Initiate IV hydration; give ethanol infusion to compete with metabolism and simultaneous dialysis for removal
OTHER CAUSES OF ALTERED MENTAL STATUS		
	(Refer to Chapter 27, Care Plan for Unresponsive Patient)	
DISULFIRAM (ANTABUSE) REACTION		
	Caused by simultaneous alcohol ingestion; reaction occurs from accumulation of acetaldehyde during alcohol metabolism; results in flushing, tachycardia, diaphoresis, nausea, vomiting, hyper- or hypotension—may occur up to 2 weeks following last dose of disulfiram	Initiate IV hydration

IMPLEMENTATION

I. Primary intervention
   A. Protect airway
      1. Severe respiratory depression warrants intubation
      2. Position patient on side to prevent aspiration
   B. Establish intravenous access
      1. If patient is obtunded: dextrose and normal saline solution TKO
      2. If patient is dehydrated: dextrose 5% normal saline or dextrose 5% lactated Ringer's 200 to 500 ml per hour
      3. Multivitamins and thiamine: 50 to 100 mg IV or IM
      4. Dextrose 50% IV push; assess need by dextrostix
   C. Evaluate other complaints or concerns of altered mental status
      1. Obtain alcohol level if patient
         a) Is obtunded
         b) Has head injury with loss of consciousness
         c) Exhibits unexplained bizarre behavior
      2. Refer to specific care plan for management guidelines
   D. Protect patient from injury
      1. Intoxicated patient's right to refuse treatment requires careful consideration if there are life- or limb-threatening injuries
      2. Employ Alcohol Hold Procedure (will vary from state to state)
         a) Instituted to prevent patient from leaving department until more sober and able to make informed decision
         b) Patient may be restrained as necessary
         c) Alcohol hold may be required for suicidal ideation
      3. Patient must be capable of ambulation before being discharged from the department

II. Secondary intervention
   A. Check serial vital signs with particular attention to mental and respiratory assessment
   B. Anticipate rate of alcohol metabolism at 10 to 30 mg %/hr
   C. If patient's mental status fails to improve, reconsider other causes of altered mental status
   D. Orient patient as arousal occurs
   E. Offer fluids and comfort measures
   F. Assess interest in detoxification program
   G. Assess patient's support system and consider possible referral to community resources

EVALUATION

I. Patient outcomes/criteria
   A. Oriented to person, place, and time
   B. Gross ataxia resolved
   C. Return of vital signs to within normal limits
   D. Decreased or resolved agitation
   E. Resolution of accompanying complaints
II. Document initial assessment data, emergency department interventio and patient's response to treatment
III. If the previous patient outcomes are not reached, the emergency nur should reevaluate the interventions and change the plan of care accor ingly

DISPOSITION

I. Admission criteria
   A. Warranted by accompanying illness or trauma
   B. Detoxification program
II. Discharge guidelines
   A. Offer alcohol counseling, if available, to patient and family
   B. Check for potential drug interactions such as antabuse, sedatives, etc

CHAPTER 3

ALCOHOL WITHDRAWAL

MPLICATIONS FOR ACTION

lcohol withdrawal produces a variety of symptoms ranging from tremors and ritability to the hallucinations of full-blown delirium tremens which, while are, one must be alert for. There may also be marked confusion and autoomic hyperactivity. Prompt recognition and treatment of the withdrawal yndrome in its early stages helps to alleviate the patient's anxiety and to prevent the development of major withdrawal patterns.

SSESSMENT

I. Initial observation
   A. Tremulousness, agitation
   B. Level of consciousness
II. Subjective assessment
   A. History from patient or family
      1. Length of current drinking episode
      2. Type of alcohol consumed per day
      3. Time of last drink
      4. History of withdrawal seizures or delirium tremens
      5. Previous detoxification methods
         a) Inpatient unit or outpatient therapy
         b) Antabuse treatment
   B. Associated symptoms
      1. Nausea and vomiting; hematemesis
      2. Grossly bloody or tarry stools
      3. Abdominal pain
      4. Irritability
      5. Hallucinations (most commonly visual, may also be audio, tactile, olfactory); confusion
      6. Weakness
      7. Insomnia

- C. Previous or concurrent medical disorders
  1. Liver disease: cirrhosis or hepatitis
  2. Coagulopathies
  3. Gastrointestinal (GI) bleeding
  4. Pancreatitis
  5. Medications and allergies

III. Objective assessment

- A. Vital signs
  1. Orthostatic blood pressure and pulse, which is often tachycardi[c,] should be obtained
  2. Respiratory rate and character
  3. Temperature
- B. Mental status
  1. Level of orientation
  2. Appropriateness of conversation
  3. Hallucinations
  4. Confusion
- C. Skin color, temperature, presence of diaphoresis
- D. Tremors, agitation, anxiety
- E. Nystagmus; unsteady gait
- F. Evidence of seizure
  1. Altered mental status
  2. Trauma to tongue
  3. Incontinence

POSSIBLE NURSING DIAGNOSES/ANALYSIS

I. Anxiety
II. Cardiac output, alteration in: decreased
III. Fluid volume deficit, potential
IV. Injury: potential for
V. Knowledge deficit (effects of alcohol)
VI. Noncompliance
VII. Nutrition, alteration in: less than body requirements
VIII. Self-concept, disturbance in: body image, self-esteem, role performanc[e,] personal identity
IX. Sensory-perceptual alteration: visual, auditory, kinesthetic, gustator[y,] tactile, olfactory
X. Sleep pattern disturbance
XI. Social isolation
XII. Thought processes, alteration in

[PL]ANNING

[I.] Priorities for care
A. Identifying severity of withdrawal
B. Fluid management
C. Agitation control
[II.] Differential management

[C]ondition	Clinical Assessment	Management
[A]LCOHOL WITHDRAWAL		
[M]inor	Onset 8-24 hours after last drink or with abrupt reduction of alcohol intake; patient may still have positive alcohol level; duration 2-10 days; patient may have irritability, tremors, insomnia, tachycardia, nausea and vomiting, anorexia or may progress to more major withdrawal pattern with hallucinations, diaphoresis, confusion	Perform IV hydration if patient is orthostatic or unable to tolerate oral fluids; use benzodiazepines (Valium, Tranxene), propranolol
[S]eizures	Chronic alcohol use lowers seizure threshold; seizures normally occur 12-48 hours after cessation of alcohol use but are rare after 96 hours; seizures are usually grand mal, rarely focal or status, and are usually limited in number to fewer than five, but status epilepticus can occur	First documented seizure needs neurological workup to rule out other etiologies; use of antiepileptic drugs is controversial with acute withdrawal; chronic therapy not recommended for alcohol withdrawal seizures; (refer to Chapter 23, Care Plan for Seizures)

Condition	Clinical Assessment	Management
Delirium Tremens	Statistically uncommon, but there is a 5%-15% mortality rate because of circulatory collapse or hyperthermia; onset 24-96 hours after cessation of alcohol use; diagnosis based on the presence of confusion, tachycardia, and fever; other symptoms observed include increased autonomic activity: extreme agitation, hypo- or hypertension, diaphoresis, dilated pupils, mydriasis, inattention, delusions, hallucinations, gross tremors, and sleeplessness	Initiate IV hydration as well as glucose and thiamine IV; institute aggressive treatment with IV benzodiazepines (chlordiazepoxide, diazepam)
Alcoholic Ketoacidosis (AKA)	Ketones are formed during metabolism of alcohol and because of impaired liver function cannot be metabolized to glucose and glycogen; there is a history of recent alcohol binge with poor nutrition; patient may have anorexia, nausea, and protracted vomiting, tachypnea, Kussmaul respirations, ketonemia, hypoglycemia, negative alcohol level, mixed acid-base disturbance, vomiting leading to metabolic alkalosis, AKA resulting in metabolic acidosis, hyperpnea resulting in respiratory alkalosis	Initiate IV hydration with dextrose or dextrose and saline (125-150 ml/hr) to correct acidosis (usually takes 12-16 hours); check electrolytes; give thiamine 100 mg IM or IV and phosphate supplement

ondition	Clinical Assessment	Management
ERNICKE-KORSAKOFF SYNDROME		
	Not a withdrawal state but occurs in chronic alcoholics with poor nutrition, caused by dietary lack of thiamine (vitamin B_1), which facilitates glucose metabolism; acute or chronic triad of signs: recent memory loss, wide-based or ataxic gait, nystagmus or ocular palsies; patient may have tachycardia, orthostatic hypotension, weakness; condition may lead to coma; there is often concomitant magnesium deficiency	Administer thiamine 100 mg IV; then 50-100 mg IV or IM q.d. until patient resumes normal diet; hydrate with dextrose and magnesium: 2 gm (50% magnesium sulfate) IM

MPLEMENTATION

. Primary intervention

A. Initiate intravenous access for hydration
   1. Monitor orthostatic vital signs; infuse dextrose and saline or dextrose and lactated Ringer's solution until rehydration is achieved
   2. Use IV if patient is unable to tolerate oral fluids
   3. Provide access for medications

B. Administer medications: as outlined in differential management section
   1. For withdrawal symptoms
      a) Chlorazepate (Tranxene): 15 to 30 mg PO q3 to 6 hours
      b) Diazepam (Valium): 2.5 to 20 mg PO, IM, or IV q4 to 6 hours
      c) Chlordiazepoxide (Librium): 25 to 100 mg IM or IV q4 to 6 hours
   2. For malnutrition
      a) Thiamine: 50 to 100 mg IM or IV; PO not absorbed well
      b) Multivitamins: usually added to IV solution; many contain thiamine
      c) Dextrose 50% IV if hypoglycemia is suspected or if indicated by dextrostix

- C. Protect patient who is markedly agitated from injury
  1. Put side rails up
  2. Restrain as necessary
  3. Decrease stimuli in environment

II. Secondary intervention
- A. Obtain laboratory data
  1. Dextrostix; hypoglycemia common in alcoholic patients
  2. Hematocrit if history is indicative of gastrointestinal bleeding
  3. Complete blood count if patient is febrile
  4. Electrolytes if AKA is suspected or patient has had prolonged vomitin
  5. Urine dipstick for ketones
- B. Consider other causes of decreased mentation (such as intracrania trauma or sepsis) (refer to Chapter 27, Care Plan for the Unresponsiv Patient)
- C. Perform serial vital signs and mental status evaluation
- D. Assess patient's interest in a detoxification program

EVALUATION

I. Patient outcomes/criteria
- A. Return to normal mentation
- B. Return of vital signs to within normal limits
- C. Decreased agitation, tremors

II. Document initial assessment data, emergency department intervention and patient's response to pharmacologic therapy

III. If previous patient outcomes are not reached, the emergency nurse shoulc reevaluate the interventions and change the plan of care accordingly

DISPOSITION

I. Admission criteria
- A. Delirium tremens
- B. Wernicke-Korsakoff syndrome
- C. Concomitant pathology (such as pneumonia, unresolved electrolyte imbalance, or gastrointestinal bleeding)
- D. Inability to tolerate oral fluids
- E. Patient may be admitted to medical unit or alcohol detoxification unit

II. Discharge guidelines
- A. Arrange outpatient counseling for patient and family if they are agree-able
- B. Provide community resource information (such as numbers for Alco-holics Anonymous, Al-Anon, 24-hour telephone crisis lines) as available

CHAPTER 4

CHEST PAIN

MPLICATIONS FOR ACTION

'he patient with chest pain requires a decisive and expeditious triage for im-
ediate evaluation because of the high incidence of complications with seri-
us cardiovascular or pulmonary sources of chest discomfort. Initial concern
volves treating life-threatening dysrhythmias and ensuring adequate oxygen-
tion. The frightening nature of this occurrence mandates a calm, reassuring
pproach to the patient and his or her family. The following protocol outlines
he priorities for care of the patient with chest pain.

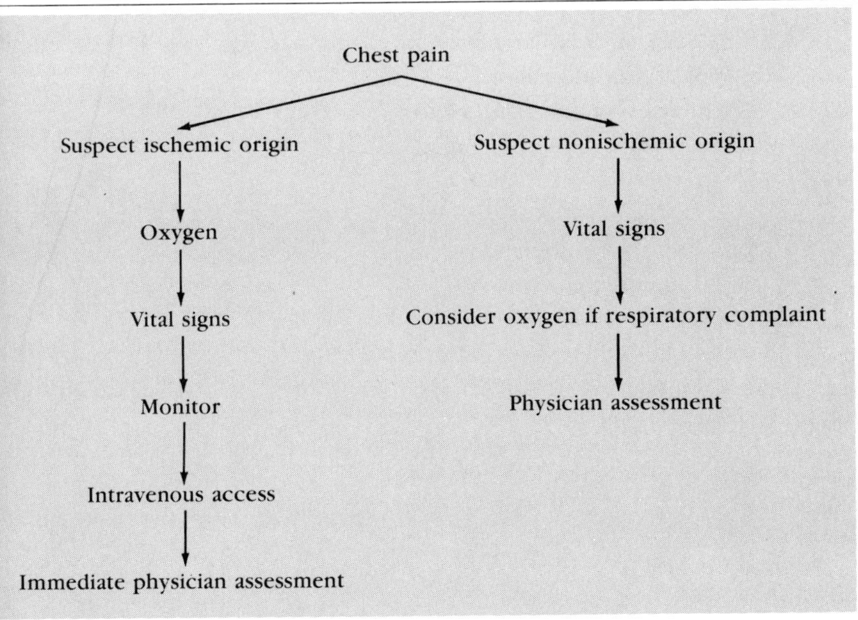

ASSESSMENT

I. Initial observation
   A. Skin color
   B. Respiratory effort
   C. Anxiety
II. Subjective assessment
   A. Description of pain
      1. Time of onset: gradual or sudden
      2. Activity at onset
      3. Location
      4. Sharp, dull, pressure-like
      5. Intermittent or constant
      6. Radiation
      7. Change in pain with deep inspiration, cough, or movement
   B. Associated symptoms
      1. Nausea, vomiting
      2. Shortness of breath
      3. Diaphoresis
      4. Cough: productive or nonproductive
      5. Fever
   C. Measures taken to relieve pain such as rest, nitroglycerine, antacids
   D. Past medical history
      1. Previous myocardial infarction, cardiac surgery
      2. Medications and allergies
      3. Presence of cardiac risk factors
         a) Smoking
         b) Hypertension
         c) Diabetes mellitus
         d) Positive family history
         e) Hypercholesterolemia
         f) Obesity
   E. Recent stress, illness, or exertional activity (if trauma is suspected cause of pain, refer to Chapter 34, Care Plan for Major Multiple Trauma)

I. Objective assessment
   A. Complete vital signs
   B. Level of consciousness may be diminished because of hypoxia, or, more rarely, hypercapnia
   C. Respiratory effort
      1. Use of accessory muscles
      2. Breath sounds
         a) Compare bilaterally
         b) Presence of rales, wheezes
      3. Heart sounds
         a) Friction rub suggests pericarditis
         b) Murmurs suggest valvular disease or endocarditis
   D. Skin color pale, cyanotic, ashen, or flushed
   E. Skin temperature warm, cool, or diaphoretic

POSSIBLE NURSING DIAGNOSES/ANALYSIS

I. Anxiety
II. Breathing pattern, ineffective
III. Cardiac output, alteration in: decreased
IV. Comfort, alteration in: pain
V. Fluid volume, alteration in: excess
VI. Gas exchange, impaired
VII. Knowledge deficit (regarding present illness)
VIII. Tissue perfusion, alteration in: cerebral, cardiopulmonary, renal, gastro-intestinal

PLANNING

I. Priorities for care
   A. Recognition and treatment of life-threatening dysrhythmias
   B. Hemodynamic stabilization
   C. Isolating cause of chest pain
   D. Relief of anxiety if possible
II. Differential management

Condition	Clinical Assessment	Management
CARDIOVASCULAR		
Myocardial Ischemia or Infarct	Substernal or left chest pain often described as crushing pain or pressure; may radiate to patient's left arm or jaw; associated symptoms include nausea, vomiting, diaphoresis, dyspnea; ECG may show ST segment elevation or depression, T wave inversion, ventricular irritability; ventricular failure may develop resulting in pulmonary (left ventricular failure) or venous (right ventricular failure) congestion, which may progress to cardiogenic shock	Establish intravenous access, give antidysrhythmics, analgesics, or nitroglycerin; perform continuous cardiac monitoring; oxygen administration 3-6 L/min via nasal prongs; admission blood work includes cardiac enzymes
Dysrhythmias	Rapid tachycardias may cause a sensation of chest pain or pounding in the chest; dysrhythmias disrupt and lead to decreased coronary perfusion resulting in ischemic pain, further compromising the oxygenation of the injured muscle	Treatment of life-threatening dysrhythmias outlined in Chapter 17, Care Plan for Medical Cardiopulmonary Arrest
Pericarditis	Inflammation of pericardial sac resulting in severe chest pain; may increase with respiration or activity; accompanying symptoms include fever, diaphoresis; dyspnea with ST elevation and pericardial rub often present; pain classically relieved by sitting forward	Oxygen 3-6 L/min via nasal prongs; give antiinflammatory agents; rest recommended

ndition	Clinical Assessment	Management
oracic Aortic ssection	Sudden tearing chest pain perceived mainly in the back and possibly abdomen; symptoms include dyspnea, diaphoresis, pallor, tachycardia, hypertension, asymmetric pulses and blood pressures, neurological deficits; widened mediastinum on chest x ray; signs and symptoms depend on location of dissection and specific arterial branches of aorta involved; pain not relieved with analgesics; rupture of dissection results in rapid exsanguination	Establish intravenous access; give antihypertensives; oxygen administration at 3-6 L/min via nasal prongs; diagnosis with angiography; often necessitates surgical repair
ULMONARY		
lmonary Embolus	Pleuritic chest pain, tachypnea, dyspnea, tachycardia, cough with hemoptysis, anxiety; higher risk factor patients are those with history of immobilization, phlebitis, long-bone fractures, or oral contraceptive use	Obtain arterial blood gases; diagnosis with lung scan or angiography; treat with streptokinase or anticoagulation; obtain baseline partial thromboplastin time and administer heparin 5-10,000 units as an intravenous bolus followed by continuous infusion
ontaneous neumothorax	Sudden onset of pleuritic chest pain and dyspnea; patient may have diminished breath sounds on affected side; most frequently occurs in young males or older patients with chronic obstructive lung disease	Diagnosis confirmed by chest x-ray study but obtaining this should not delay treatment for severe respiratory distress; treat with chest tube insertion if indicated by size of pneumothorax or symptoms (refer to appendix A for procedure and equipment)

Condition	Clinical Assessment	Management
Pneumonia	Pleuritic chest pain often accompanied by fever, cough, malaise; patient may have history of recent respiratory tract illness	Obtain complete blood count and sputum cultures; diagnosis is confirmed by chest x-ray study; treat with antibiotics, oxygen and fluids; elderly or debilitated patients may require admission
Pleurisy	Sharp chest pain, increases with inspiration; may involve infectious process resulting in fever and dyspnea	Treat with rest, antiinflammatory agents, possibly antibiotics
MUSCULOSKELETAL		
	Caused by inflammation of muscles, bones, joints, muscular spasm or strain, or rib fractures; localized, point tender pain, increases with movement; usually without dyspnea; patient may have history of recent trauma or exertional activity	Rest; administer antiinflammatory agents; (refer to Chapter 34, Care Plan for Major Multiple Trauma)
HYPERVENTILATION SYNDROME		
	Rapid shallow breathing resulting in respiratory alkalosis; circumoral and peripheral paresthesias, carpopedal spasm; must be sure symptoms are not due to underlying disorder such as compensation for acidosis, fever, pulmonary or neurological disorder, hypovolemia	If anxiety is the cause, use calm approach to patient with reassurance; if necessary have patient rebreathe into small paper bag; insert or use an oxygen rebreather mask with holes taped closed; treat underlying pathology if present
OTHER CAUSES		
	Abdominal disorders may elicit chest pain	(Refer to Chapter 1, Care Plan for Abdominal Pain)

IPLEMENTATION

Primary intervention

A. Obtain intravenous access
   1. When cardiac origin suspected
   2. If patient exhibits respiratory distress or cyanosis
   3. Infuse dextrose 5% with microdrip at TKO rate to avoid fluid overload
B. Institute cardiac monitoring
   1. Continuous bedside monitoring with lead MCL or lead II
   2. Obtain 12-lead ECG
C. Administer oxygen
   1. 3 to 6 L/min via nasal prongs; consider lower flow rate for patients with chronic obstructive pulmonary disease
   2. Do not withhold oxygen to obtain arterial blood gases if patient is in respiratory distress
D. Administer medications
   1. Antidysrhythmics
      a) Lidocaine: 50 to 100 mg intravenous bolus over several minutes, followed by infusion of 2 to 4 mg/min; repeat bolus one half of original dose in 10 minutes
      b) Refer to Chapter 17, Care Plan for Medical Cardiopulmonary Arrest
   2. Nitroglycerin
      a) Commonly used to treat angina or ischemic pain
      b) Sublingual, intravenous, or dermal route
      c) Following administration, blood pressure should be monitored as hypotension can develop regardless of route
   3. Analgesia: morphine 2 to 4 mg intravenous boluses for relief of severe pain
   4. Heparin according to hospital protocol
E. Laboratory data as outlined in differential management section

Secondary intervention

A. Position head of bed for patient's comfort; should be flat if patient is hypotensive
B. Determine serial vital signs
C. Provide continuous cardiac monitoring if dysrhythmias present
D. Explain treatment to patient and family to diminish anxiety

EVALUATION

I. Patient outcomes/criteria
   A. Relief of chest pain
   B. Resolution of dysrhythmias
   C. Absence of respiratory distress
   D. Diminished anxiety

II. Document initial assessment data, emergency department interventio and patient's response to treatment

III. If previous patient outcomes are not reached, the emergency nurse shoul reevaluate the interventions and change the plan of care accordingly

DISPOSITION

I. Admission criteria
   A. New onset or unstable angina, evolving myocardial infarction, vascula aneurysm, congestive failure, dysrhythmias, or unresolved pain
   B. Pulmonary embolus, pneumothorax, pneumonia requiring intravenou antibiotics or supportive therapy

II. Discharge guidelines
   A. Give instructions concerning cause of pain
   B. Make follow-up arrangements as appropriate
   C. Give medication instructions

CHAPTER 5

CHILDBIRTH: EMERGENCY DELIVERY

IPLICATIONS FOR ACTION

ais care plan is designed to offer direction in the case of an emergency deliv-y. Chapter 28, Care Plan for Vaginal Bleeding, also includes a discussion of mplications of pregnancy. The two most important items to remember dur-g a delivery are:

1. Airway management of the infant
2. Control of bleeding in the mother

SSESSMENT

I. Initial observation
   A. Emotional status of mother
   B. Obvious rupture of membranes (soaked clothes)
I. Subjective assessment
   A. Current status
      1. Frequency, duration, and intensity of contractions
      2. Time of onset of labor
      3. Intact or suspected rupture of membranes
   B. Obstetrical history
      1. Gravida, parity
      2. Estimated due date
      3. Prenatal care
      4. Complications during pregnancy
      5. Medications and allergies
I. Objective assessment
   A. Vital signs, if time available
      1. Fetal heart tones
      2. Mother: blood pressure, pulse, respirations

B. Relevant status
  1. Character and amount of show
  2. Bulging perineum
  3. Appearance of presenting part if crowning
  4. Involuntary pushing indicative of imminent delivery

POSSIBLE NURSING DIAGNOSES/ANALYSIS

I. Airway clearance, ineffective (newborn)
II. Anxiety
III. Comfort, alteration in: pain
IV. Knowledge deficit (of the birth event)
V. Tissue perfusion, alteration in: peripheral

PLANNING

I. Priorities for care
  A. Recognition of imminent delivery
  B. During labor assist mother in gaining emotional control
  C. During delivery
    1. Manage infant's airway
    2. Control speed of delivery to prevent complications to mother an infant
    3. Control maternal blood loss
II. Review of mechanism of labor
  A. Descent: associated with various movements of the fetus as it passe through the birth canal
  B. Engagement: the widest diameter of fetus's head is at or passes the pelvic inlet
  C. Flexion: neck is flexed with chin touching sternum to allow presentation of smaller diameter
  D. Internal rotation: head rotates on shoulders to pass through narrow diameter of pelvis
  E. Extension: occiput of infant's head is born; mother's pelvic arch acts a pivotal point on neck allowing extension of head and presentation o face
  F. Restitution and external rotation: infant's head turns to face mother's thigh; shoulders rotate to anterior/posterior diameter of pelvis
  G. Positions may be altered because of child's presentation

MPLEMENTATION

. Primary intervention

A. Delivery

1. Convey calmness and help mother focus attention on delivery and your voice
2. Obtain quick history if time permits
3. Position mother in bed (if possible) with head elevated; she may be more comfortable on side
4. Instruct mother to pant or blow through contractions
5. Send available person for supplies and assistance; precipitous delivery pack should include bulb syringe, towels or blanket, sterile scissors, and two clamps; if available use sterile gloves and DeLee suction (refer to appendix A for equipment tray)
6. As infant's head becomes more visible, control the advancement with gentle pressure of one hand; once head is delivered, wipe or suction secretions from infant's mouth and nose; if meconium is present, suction nose and mouth with DeLee suction
7. Check if cord is wrapped around baby's neck; if it is tight, pull gently to loosen or slip over head; if unable to loosen cord, double clamp and cut cord
8. External rotation will occur; place hands over infant's ears and gently apply downward traction to allow delivery of anterior shoulder
9. Apply upward traction to assist delivery of posterior shoulder
10. Carefully support infant's body as it emerges; hold infant's head lower than body and place on mother's abdomen to promote drainage of secretions and to stimulate mother's uterine contractions

B. Immediate care of newborn

1. Airway management
   a) Suction mouth and nose with bulb syringe
   b) If no spontaneous cry
      (1) Gently stimulate by rubbing back or feet
      (2) Stroke trachea (toward chin) while keeping newborn's head low
   c) Give oxygen if infant is cyanotic or in respiratory distress
2. Prevent hypothermia
   a) Place newborn on mother's abdomen or allow it to suckle; this will assist in placenta/separation and delivery
   b) Cover infant with warm blanket, including head

3. Double clamp the cord with sterile equipment 3 to 5 inches fro umbilicus
4. Cut cord with sterile scissors after pulsations have ceased

C. Delivery of the placenta
1. Placental separation indicated by
a) Sudden gush of blood
b) Lengthening of cord
2. Lift the cord and placenta as it is delivered during contractio DO NOT PULL ON CORD!
3. Massage the fundus with gentle circular strokes to control bleedin
4. Initiate intravenous line of 0.9 normal saline or lactated Ringer's bleeding continues

II. Secondary intervention
A. Maintain supportive atmosphere for mother and family
B. Use calm voice, eye contact, and touch to alleviate fear and anxiety
C. Provide comfort measures when possible
D. Repeat uterine massage to help prevent excessive bleeding

EVALUATION

I. Patient outcomes: mother
A. Perineum should be assessed for hematoma or lacerations
B. Firm fundus to palpation
C. Minimal bleeding
D. Normal vital signs

II. Patient outcomes: newborn
A. Patent airway without respiratory distress
B. Pink skin color
C. Assess Apgar score at 1 and 5 minutes (refer to table on opposite page)

III. Document initial assessment of emergency delivery course and conditio of mother and newborn after delivery

IV. If previous patient outcomes are not reached, the emergency nurse shoul reevaluate the interventions and change the plan of care accordingly

DISPOSITION

I. Transport mother and newborn to appropriate unit in the hospital
II. Nurse or physician should accompany the patients

pgar Score

	0	1	2
eart rate	Absent	<100	>100
espirations	Absent	Slow, irregular	Good, crying
uscle tone	Flaccid	Some flexion of extremities	Active motion
eflex irritability	No response	Weak cry or grimace	Vigorous cry
olor	Blue, pale	Body pink, extremities blue	Completely pink

ORE: 7-10 Good
4-6 Fair: clear airway, give oxygen
0-3 Poor: requires resuscitation efforts

CHAPTER 6

DIABETIC EMERGENCIES: ALTERATIONS IN BLOOD GLUCOSE

IMPLICATIONS FOR ACTION

The diabetic patient entering the emergency department may exhibit a varie of symptoms. Rapid clinical assessment quickly isolates life-threatening hyp or hyperglycemia. These conditions should always be considered when ev uating the unresponsive patient.

The diabetic patient is more prone to "silent" myocardial infarctions (M with minimal pain. Because of the high incidence of complications, a history diabetes is significant even when the patient enters with an unrelated illness injury.

ASSESSMENT

I. Initial observation
   A. Skin color
   B. Respiratory status
   C. Level of consciousness
II. Subjective assessment
   A. History of diabetes
      1. Insulin-dependent; diet or oral hypoglycemic agent–controlled
         a) Compliance with medication and diet
         b) Recent change in medication dosage
      2. Duration of disease and degree of control
      3. Complications of diabetes such as retinopathy, peripheral neuro athy, renal disease
   B. Associated symptoms
      1. Hunger
      2. Polyuria, polydipsia

3. Gastrointestinal complaints: nausea, vomiting, diarrhea, abdominal pain
4. Dizziness, weakness, syncope
5. Restlessness, anxiety, nervousness
6. Infectious symptoms of the throat, ear, chest, urinary tract

C. Recent stress: physical or psychological

I. Objective assessment

A. Vital signs
1. Blood pressure, pulse: unless hypotensive (systolic BP <90)
2. Respiratory rate and character
    a) Kussmaul breathing (rapid, deep): respiratory response to metabolic acidosis—pH <7.2
    b) Fruity, acetone odor of breath indicative of ketoacidosis; may be difficult to detect
3. Temperature: an infection often precipitates decompensation; temperature may be normal or decreased in diabetic ketoacidosis (DKA) even with infection

B. Altered mental status ranging from lethargy or stupor to coma

C. Signs of dehydration
1. Dry skin and mucous membranes
2. Decreased skin turgor
3. Orthostatic dizziness
4. Thirst, tachycardia, hypotension

D. Pallor

E. Diaphoresis

F. Shaking, tremor

OSSIBLE NURSING DIAGNOSES/ANALYSIS

I. Airway clearance, ineffective
II. Breathing pattern, ineffective
III. Cardiac output, alteration in: decreased
IV. Fluid volume deficit, actual
V. Gas exchange, impaired
VI. Knowledge deficit (diabetes)
VII. Noncompliance
III. Nutrition, alteration in: less than and more than body requirements
IX. Skin integrity, impairment of: potential
X. Thought processes, alteration in
XI. Tissue perfusion, alteration in: cerebral, renal, peripheral
XII. Urinary elimination, alteration in patterns

PLANNING

I. Priorities for care
   A. Airway management
   B. Fluid management
   C. Serum electrolyte to include acid/base balance
   D. Glucose management
II. Differential management

Condition	Clinical Assessment	Management
HYPOGLYCEMIA		
	Occurs in patients with diabetes, usually the result of too much insulin or oral hypoglycemic as the usual agent; or with the usual dose from a failure to eat or because of increased exercise; symptoms include hunger, anxiety, restlessness, diaphoresis, dilated pupils, weakness, headache; patient may have seizures progressing to coma or rapid development of symptoms and deterioration in condition	Assess with dextrostix and glucose; rapid improvement occurs with 50% glucose bolus IV; if severe hypoglycemia occurs in the nondiabetic patient, other causes such as endocrinopathies or pancreatic tumor must be co sidered; patient may require prolonged observation if ove dose is suspected (refer to insulin preparation chart at end of care plan for when th insulin will peak); patient ma require multiple boluses of dextrose 50% to reverse hypoglycemia
HYPERGLYCEMIC HYPEROSMOLAR NONKETOTIC COMA (HHNKC)		
	Generally occurs in mild or undiagnosed diabetic patients in their 60s or 70s; characterized by hyperglycemia, dehydration, and coma without acidosis or ketonemia (mild acidosis may be present); patient may have grand mal seizures	40%-70% mortality without ea aggressive management; trea ment similar to DKA with hydration and potassium supplementation; usually patient should be rehydrated le rapidly than in DKA; obtain glucose and electrolyte measurements; monitor urinary output; complications includ cerebral edema, pulmonary edema, thrombophlebitis, car diac dysrhythmias, electrolyte disturbances, urinary tra infection

ondition	Clinical Assessment	Management
IABETIC KETOACIDOSIS (DKA)		
	Results from insulin depletion because of noncompliance or increased demand; develops over 36-48 hours; failure of glucose to enter cells to be metabolized causes it to act as an osmotic; glucose is an osmotic diuretic and causes water loss accompanied by sodium and potassium loss, resulting in hypovolemia and electrolyte imbalance; protein and fat are used for metabolic energy requirements, increasing plasma concentrations of amino acids and free fatty acids, resulting in acidosis; patient may have dehydration, orthostasis, nausea, vomiting, abdominal pain, rapid deep breathing (Kussmaul respirations), acetone odor on breath, possibly altered mental status	Initiate IV hydration with normal or half normal saline; give potassium supplement, regular insulin: IV bolus and infusion, possibly sodium bicarbonate; obtain laboratory data: dextrostix, glucose, electrolytes, arterial blood gases to determine acidosis, complete blood count to rule out systemic infection, ECG in patients 40 years or older ("silent" myocardial infarction [MI] may be precipitated by DKA); ECG to determine hypo- or hyperkalemia, urine dipstick for ketones and glucose, urinalysis to rule out urinary tract infection, serial electrolyte and glucose measurements
LCOHOLIC KETOACIDOSIS (AKA)		
	Occurs in patient during alcohol metabolism; ketones are formed; patient may have anorexia, nausea, vomiting, abdominal pain, tachycardia, tachypnea, Kussmaul respirations; laboratory studies usually indicate a low to normal glucose level, ketonemia, and acidosis	Initiate IV hydration with dextrose and saline to correct acidosis; treat volume deficits, administer thiamine 100 mg IV or IM, potassium supplements (refer to Chapter 3, Care Plan for Alcohol Withdrawal)

IMPLEMENTATION

I. Primary intervention
   A. Establish airway management
      1. Comatose patient may require intubation
      2. Oxygen at 2 to 6 L/min via prongs or mask
   B. Initiate intravenous hydration
      1. Start one or two large-bore peripheral IVs; central venous pressu (CVP) line may be inserted if patient is hypotensive
      2. If DKA or AKA is suspected, infuse normal saline
         a) In adults: 100 to 200 ml rapid infusion, then 200 to 500 ml/hou
         b) In children: 20 ml/kg over 30 min, then may repeat 10 ml/ followed by 100 to 200 ml/hour
   C. Give medications: refer to differential management section for guic lines
      1. Glucose 50% (dextrose 50%) 25 gm IV and naloxone 0.8-1.6 mg as indicated for the unresponsive patient
         a) Hypoglycemic patient may respond dramatically to a single bolus of dextrose 50% but may also require several boluses
         b) Use dextrostix to determine necessity of dextrose 50%
         c) In children up to age 3—2 to 4 ml dextrose 25%/kg
      2. Insulin
         a) Use only regular insulin for IV doses
         b) Give regular insulin, usually 5 to 10 units IV push initially
         c) Insulin infusion will be ordered at a specific number of unit hour
            (1) Refer to chart at end of care plan for concentration and c culation of rates
            (2) Mix in normal saline
            (3) Flush IV tubing with 20 to 30 ml of solution as initial insul may adhere to tubing
            (4) Infusion for adults initially 5 to 10 units/hour; children 0 unit/kg/hour
            (5) Maintain accuracy of drip with infusion pump
      3. Potassium
         a) Total body stores of potassium depleted because of diures vomiting, and shifts with acidosis
         b) Because of acidosis and dehydration, initial serum potassium normal or elevated in majority of cases

   c) Serum potassium drops rapidly in first 4 hours of treatment with insulin infusion and correction of acidosis
   d) Potassium phosphate should be added to IV solution; cardiac monitor should be used if rate is 10 mEq/hour or greater
4. Sodium bicarbonate
   a) Usually not given unless pH is less than 7.0; acidosis corrects with hydration and insulin
   b) Administration, if ordered, 1 to 2 ampules IV (44 mEq/ampule) push and 1 ampule added to IV solution

D. Obtain laboratory data
1. Indicated in differential management section
2. Dextrostix
   a) Quickly performed in emergency department
   b) Accurately indicates hypoglycemia
   c) Estimates extent of hyperglycemia
   d) Elderly persons may falsely show hypoglycemia

Secondary intervention

A. Insert indwelling urinary catheter for accurate record of intake and output
B. Serially monitor vital signs, serum glucose and electrolytes, and mental status
C. Diagnose and treat underlying disease or precipitating factors
1. Infection
2. Nausea, vomiting
3. Noncompliance
4. Stress
5. Chronic disease
6. Concurrent medications

ALUATION

Patient outcomes/criteria

A. Normal vital signs; resolution of orthostasis
B. Correction of glucose and electrolyte imbalances
C. Improved mental status

Document initial assessment data, emergency department intervention, and patient's response to treatment

If previous patient outcomes are not reached, the emergency nurse should reevaluate the interventions and change the plan of care accordingly

DISPOSITION

I. Admission criteria
   A. Overdoses of insulin preparations or oral hypoglycemic agents that h: an extended duration of action
   B. Patient's serum glucose remains above 300 or patient continues to acidotic
   C. Patient unable to tolerate oral fluids
   D. Precipitating cause is uncorrected or patient needs hospital mana ment
   E. Many patients will clear within 6 to 12 hours of treatment and can successfully managed in the emergency department

II. Discharge guidelines
   A. Begin patient and family teaching concerning
      1. Diet and medication interaction
      2. Times of peak action of medications (refer to tables at end of t care plan)
      3. Obtaining prompt medical attention when ill
   B. Arrange follow-up care

Insulin Preparation Chart

Category	Type	Onset	Peak	Durati
Rapid acting	Regular	IV: immed	15-30 min	2 hrs
		SQ: 30-60 min	2-6 hrs	6-10 h
		IM: 5-30 min	30-60 min	2-4 hr
	Semilente	SQ: 30-60 min	2-6 hrs	8-16 h
Intermediate acting	NPH Iletin	SQ: 1-3 hrs	6-12 hrs	12-14
	Lente	SQ: 1-3 hrs	6-12 hrs	14-28
Slow acting	Protamine, zinc (PZI)	SQ: 4-6 hrs	14-20 hrs	24-36
	Ultralente	SQ: 4-6 hrs	18 hrs	24-36

ral Hypoglycemic Agents

ype	Peak	Duration
cetohexamide (Dymelor)	3-4 hours	12-24 hours
hlorpropamide (Diabinese)	2-4 hours	Up to 72 hours
olazamide (Tolinase)	4-8 hours	12-24 hours
olbutamide (Orinase)	5-8 hours	6-12 hours

nsulin Infusion Chart

oncentration	Rate	Dilution
unit/5 ml	1u/hour = 5 ml/hour	50 units regular insulin in 250 ml normal saline or 100 units regular insulin in 500 ml normal saline
	2u/hour = 10 ml/hour	
	3u/hour = 15 ml/hour	
	4u/hour = 20 ml/hour	
	5u/hour = 25 ml/hour	
	6u/hour = 30 ml/hour	
	7u/hour = 35 ml/hour	
	8u/hour = 40 ml/hour	
	9u/hour = 45 ml/hour	
	10u/hour = 50 ml/hour	
unit/10 ml	1u/hour = 10 ml/hour	50 units regular insulin in 500 ml normal saline or 100 units regular insulin in 1000 ml normal saline
	2u/hour = 20 ml/hour	
	3u/hour = 30 ml/hour	
	4u/hour = 40 ml/hour	
	5u/hour = 50 ml/hour	
	6u/hour = 60 ml/hour	
	7u/hour = 70 ml/hour	
	8u/hour = 80 ml/hour	
	9u/hour = 90 ml/hour	
	10u/hour = 100 ml/hour	

CHAPTER 7

DYSURIA

IMPLICATIONS FOR ACTION

Dysuria is a common symptom of patients entering the emergency depa ment. A detailed history will elicit the information required for appropria intervention.

ASSESSMENT

I. Initial observation
   A. Skin color
   B. Body positioning when patient is ambulatory and lying down
II. Subjective assessment
   A. History
      1. Onset and location of pain
      2. Burning, frequency, urgency, hematuria
      3. Inability to void or empty bladder completely
      4. Difficulty starting stream
      5. Trauma, previous urinary tract infection, or other genitourina problems
      6. Discharge
      7. Associated symptoms: fever, chills, malaise, nausea, vomiting
      8. Date of last menstrual period
   B. Allergies, current medications
III. Objective assessment
   A. Vital signs
      1. Fever is indicative of systemic infection; characteristic of pyel nephritis, not cystitis
      2. Orthostatic vital signs should be obtained if history is indicative dehydration
   B. Skin condition
      1. Color
      2. Diaphoresis

C. Acuteness of discomfort
   1. CVA tenderness
   2. Distention

POSSIBLE NURSING DIAGNOSES/ANALYSIS

I. Comfort, alteration in: pain
II. Fluid volume deficit: actual or potential
III. Knowledge deficit (of urinary infections)
IV. Urinary elimination, alteration in patterns

PLANNING

I. Priorities for care
   A. Hydration
   B. Other causes of abdominal discomfort should be ruled out (refer to Chapter 1, Care Plan for Abdominal Pain)
II. Differential management

Condition	Clinical Assessment	Management
LOWER TRACT INFECTION		
	Frequency, urgency, dysuria, lower abdominal (suprapubic) pain; patient may have hematuria	Patient usually treated as outpatient with antibiotics and possibly antispasmodics
UPPER TRACT INFECTION		
	Fever, chills, malaise, flank pain or costovertebral angle tenderness; possibly epigastric tenderness; anorexia, occasionally nausea and vomiting	Antibiotics and antispasmodics; patient may be treated as inpatient for IV medications and hydration
URINARY TRACT CALCULUS		
	Excruciating, intermittent pain; patient may have inability to void (obstruction) or decrease in pain after voiding (stone passed); may be accompanied by an infection secondary to obstruction and reflux	Hydration; intravenous pyelogram

Condition	Clinical Assessment	Management
URINARY RETENTION		
	Distinguish inability to void from hesitancy of lower urinary tract infection; lower abdominal pain with distended bladder; possible causes: prostatitis or post-prostatectomy	Straight catheterization after voiding to check residual urin or insertion of an indwelling urinary catheter; genitourinary consult
HEMATURIA		
	Painful hematuria, usually indicative of inflammatory process; other causes: trauma, anticoagulant therapy, blood dyscrasia, tumor	Treat cause as appropriate
SEXUALLY TRANSMITTED DISEASES IN MALES		
	Burning, discharge, dysuria	Rule out urinary tract infection; confirm gonorrhea and treat with 4.8 million units of procaine penicillin

IMPLEMENTATION

I. Primary intervention
   A. Initiate IV of normal saline or lactated Ringer's if patient is orthostatic c stone obstruction is suspected
   B. Obtain urinalysis
      1. Clean catch or catheterized specimen for routine urinalysis
      2. Specimen for culture and sensitivity
   C. CBC not helpful or necessary unless temperature is elevated (excep tion: elderly patient with suspected pyelonephritis or sepsis may nc have elevated temperature)
   D. Gram stain and culture in males with discharge to rule out gonorrhe
II. Secondary intervention
   A. Administer medications
      1. Antibiotics for 7 to 10 days
         a) Give initial dose(s) IV if patient unable to tolerate oral medic tion

b) Commonly prescribed drugs
   (1) Ampicillin: 500 mg q.i.d. (if allergic to tetracycline)
   (2) Timethoprine with sulfamethoxazole (Bactrim and Septra): calculated according to body weight
   (3) Tetracycline: 500 mg q.i.d.
   (4) Macrodantin: 50 mg q.i.d.
   (5) Sulfisoxazole (Gantrisin): 2 gm initially, then 500 mg t.i.d.
   (6) Keflex: 500 mg q.i.d. (if allergic to ampicillin)

2. Antispasmodics (e.g., pyridium)
3. Analgesia for renal calculi: meperidine, 50 to 75 mg IM or IV

B. Prepare patient for intravenous pyelogram to rule out ureteral obstruction
C. Strain urine to check for passing of stone

VALUATION

I. Patient outcomes/criteria
   A. Resolution of orthostasis
   B. Relief or decrease of symptoms
   C. Follow-up urine cultures
      1. Takes 24 to 48 hours to complete culture
      2. Positive culture indicated by >100,000 organisms
      3. Check sensitivity for appropriateness of prescribed antibiotic

I. Document initial assessment data, emergency department intervention, and patient's response to treatment

I. If previous patient outcomes are not reached, the emergency nurse should reevaluate the interventions and change the plan of care accordingly

ISPOSITION

Admission criteria
   A. When continued IV antibiotics indicated (pyelonephritis or patient unable to tolerate oral medications)

Discharge instructions
   A. Emphasize importance of medication compliance
   B. Instruct patient to return if symptoms not relieved in 2 to 3 days
   C. Review with patient discharge instruction sheet, urinary tract infections sheet, or other appropriate instructions as indicated in appendix E

CHAPTER 8

EAR, NOSE, AND THROAT COMPLAINTS

IMPLICATIONS FOR ACTION

A patient who comes to the emergency department complaining of difficul swallowing or who is drooling may be an acute emergency since swelling m occlude the airway. Prepare for intubation and notify the physician imme ately. An astute emergency nurse approaches each patient with a sore thro with a certain degree of caution. Recognition and analysis of abnormal vi signs may be early indicators of those patients who are at risk for serious ness.

ASSESSMENT

I. Initial observation
   A. Respiratory status such as labored respirations, stridor
   B. Skin color
II. Subjective assessment
   A. History of present complaint, onset, and duration of symptoms
   B. Alterations in hearing or swallowing; respiratory distress
   C. Location of pain and quality
   D. Pertinent medical history
      1. Previous ear, nose, and throat (ENT) disorders or diseases
      2. History of recent upper respiratory tract infections (URI), as the are frequently associated, or recent surgeries
      3. Other pertinent past medical problems
      4. Medications and allergies
   E. History of any associated loss of consciousness or vertigo
   F. Risk factors: history of flying, diving, occupational noise exposure, de tal work

II. Objective assessment
   A. Complete vital signs—expect elevations of temperature with infectious processes
   B. Respiratory status
      1. Listen carefully for noisy breathing
      2. Look for use of any accessory muscles
      3. Observe for drooling
   C. Neurological status
      1. Level of consciousness
   D. Physical assessment
      1. Pain or tenderness in area involved
      2. Drainage from nose or ear—note characteristics: purulent, clear, bloody
      3. Change in voice
   E. Auditory assessment: check gross hearing by using watch, tuning fork, or snap of breaking applicator stick

POSSIBLE NURSING DIAGNOSES/ANALYSIS

I. Airway clearance, ineffective
II. Anxiety
III. Breathing pattern, ineffective
IV. Comfort, alteration in: pain

PLANNING

I. Priorities for care
   A. Control and maintenance of airway, breathing, and circulation (ABCs)
   B. Relief of pain
   C. Relief of anxiety
II. Differential management

Condition	Clinical Assessment	Management
EAR		
Otitis Externa or Swimmer's Ear	One of commonest ear infections; mild itching, pain, swelling, purulent discharge; movement of ear is painful	Clean debris gently from canal; instill antibiotic anti-inflammatory drops; patient teaching should emphasize environment and personal hygiene

Condition	Clinical Assessment	Management
Acute Otitis Media	Common in children; bulging tympanic membrane, fever; child often pulls at ears; feeling of fullness in ear; patient may have decreased hearing or tinnitus in affected ear	Amoxicillin × 10 days for children <10; penicillin × 10 days for children older than 12 years; application of local heat for pai analgesia
Mastoiditis	Low-grade fever, ear pain, and swelling behind ear; tenderness over mastoid process	Provide intravenous antibiotics; patients usually ad mitted
NOSE		
Rhinitis	Patient complains of stuffy, runny nose, sneezing, or epistaxis; associated other cold symptoms	Over-the-counter drugs to re lieve symptoms
Sinusitis	Headache, facial pain, or fullness; maxillary sinusitis presents as pain in adjacent face or teeth; purulent drainage from nose or to back of throat	Bed rest; humidified air; aspirin; warm compresses; if purulent superinfection occurs, administer oral or parenteral antibiotics
THROAT		
Sore Throat		
Viral	Associated with fever, malaise, myalgias	Bed rest; fluids; throat cultur
Strep	Abrupt development; dysphagia and rapid rise in fever; patient may have diffuse erythematous rash	Throat culture; bed rest; fluids; antibiotics
Peritonsillar Abscess	History of sore throat lasting 5-10 days, swollen cervical lymph node, drooling, foul breath, fever, chills, and pain with swallowing; deviated uvula	Oxygen via nasal cannula; analgesics as ordered; thro culture; obtain intravenous access; give antibiotics
TOOTHACHE		
	Pain, swelling	Analgesics; referral to dentist

MPLEMENTATION

Primary intervention
   A. Control and maintain airway
   B. Follow guidelines in differential management section
   C. Obtain intravenous access according to vital signs and hydration status
   D. Prepare patient for x rays as ordered by physician
   E. If infectious process is suspected, isolate patient from main flow of emergency department

. Secondary intervention
   A. Relieve patient's anxiety
   B. Administer medications (as determined by physician)
      1. Analgesics
      2. Antibiotics
      3. Cultures as ordered

VALUATION

I. Patient outcomes/criteria
   A. Improved respiratory status
   B. Relief of anxiety
   C. Relief of pain
   D. Return to normothermia

I. Document initial assessment data, emergency department intervention, and the patient's response to treatment

I. If previous patient outcomes are not reached, the emergency nurse should reevaluate the interventions and change the plan of care accordingly

ISPOSITION

. Admission criteria
   A. Severe dehydration and elevated temperature, especially in children
   B. Respiratory distress
   C. Infectious process requiring parenteral antibiotics
   D. Peritonsillar abscess for incision and drainage

. Discharge guidelines
   A. Explain the disease process to patient and family, including what should be expected as it progresses
   B. Give patient instructions
      1. Per physician regarding activity and follow-up
      2. Regarding medications, application, and purpose
      3. Review instruction sheets given to patient
   C. Recommend follow-up at appropriate clinic or with private physician

CHAPTER 9

EPISTAXIS

IMPLICATIONS FOR ACTION

Epistaxis is an ENT disorder commonly treated in the emergency departmen Most frequently, the bleeding site is anterior and easily controlled withou complications. Bleeding from posterior sites or because of coagulopathies i more difficult to contain and significant blood loss may occur. Intervention involve maintaining the airway and hemostasis while using a calm, reassurin approach with the patient.

ASSESSMENT

I. Initial observation
   A. Current bleeding
   B. Skin color
II. Subjective assessment
   A. Description of episode
      1. Duration and frequency of bleeding
      2. Estimated blood loss
      3. Precipitating factor such as picking nose, trauma
      4. Measures taken to stop bleeding
   B. Past medical history
      1. Previous epistaxis
      2. Recent nasal trauma, foreign body penetration
      3. Clotting disorder, liver disease, or hypertension
      4. Medications, especially anticoagulants
III. Objective assessment
   A. Vital signs; obtain orthostatic vital signs if there is history of significan blood loss or patient is dizzy or tachycardic
   B. Amount of current bleeding
   C. Respiratory difficulty
      1. Because of nasal obstruction by clot
      2. Inability to clear secretions
      3. Anxiety

D. Associated symptoms
    1. Restlessness, dizziness, syncope
    2. Nausea and hematemesis usually because of swallowed blood

)SSIBLE NURSING DIAGNOSES/ANALYSIS

I. Airway clearance, ineffective
I. Anxiety
I. Cardiac output, alteration in: decreased
'. Fluid volume deficit, potential
/. Knowledge deficit (of nose bleeds)
I. Tissue perfusion, alteration in: peripheral, cerebral

.ANNING

Priorities for care
A. Airway maintenance
B. Blood loss control
C. Hydration

IPLEMENTATION

Primary intervention
A. Maintain airway
    1. Have patient sitting, leaning slightly forward
    2. Suction if patient is unable to control secretions
    3. Encourage patient to expectorate rather than swallow blood
B. Control bleeding
    1. Pinch nose over septal cartilage
    2. Maintain pressure for minimum of 10 minutes
    3. Instruct patient to breathe through mouth
C. Hydration
    1. Obtain intravenous access if patient is orthostatic, symptomatic, or has copious blood loss
    2. Infuse lactated Ringer's or normal saline 200 to 500 ml/hour, using slower rate for elderly patients until bleeding is controlled or vital signs are normal

. Secondary intervention
A. Obtain laboratory data
    1. Perform baseline hematocrit
    2. Coagulation studies (PT/PTT and platelet count) and complete blood count if there is
        a) History of frequent recurrent epistaxis

b) Known or suspected clotting disorder
c) Patient is receiving anticoagulation therapy
3. Type and crossmatch two units of packed RBC for hematocrit le than 30%

B. Ensure specific management of bleeding site
1. Performed by physician
2. Supplies necessary to identify site of bleeding
a) Bright light
b) Suction
c) Nasal speculum and forceps
d) Gauze
3. Cauterization usually with 10% silver nitrate sticks
4. Packing materials (used if bleeding continues after cauterization)
a) Vaseline gauze
b) Hemostatic material such as Gelfoam or Surgigel
c) Nasal balloon or indwelling urinary catheter
5. Local vasoconstrictors
a) 4% to 10% cocaine
b) 1% tetracaine
c) 4% xylocaine

C. Transfuse blood or fresh frozen plasma if ordered

D. Conduct serial assessment
1. Monitor vital signs
2. Check for continued or recurrent bleeding
3. Repeat hematocrit if bleeding continues

E. Institute comfort measures
1. Use calm approach with the patient
2. Provide tissues; also water for rinsing mouth

EVALUATION

I. Patient outcomes/criteria
A. Cessation of bleeding
B. Resolution of orthostasis

II. Document initial assessment data, emergency department interventio and patient's response to treatment

III. If previous patient outcomes are not reached, the emergency nurse shoul reevaluate the interventions and change the plan of care accordingly

ISPOSITION

. Admission criteria

A. Patients with posterior packing or bilateral anterior packing

B. Active coagulopathy

C. Patients requiring blood or fresh frozen plasma transfusions

D. Patients with recurrent or persistent hemorrhage

E. Elderly patients under consideration for a vascular ligation

. Discharge guidelines

A. Arrange follow-up

1. If nasal packing applied
2. If underlying disorder requires treatment

B. Give patient specific instructions

1. Avoid forceful nose blowing
2. Open mouth when sneezing
3. Use vaseline on nares for moisture
4. Increase home humidity
5. In case of epistaxis at home:
   a) Sit forward and pinch nose for 10 minutes
   b) If bleeding is not controlled, return to hospital
6. Do not pick clots from nose

CHAPTER 10

EYE COMPLAINTS

IMPLICATIONS FOR ACTION

A patient who comes to the emergency department with sudden painless unilateral vision loss is a true emergency. This is a sign of central retinal arter occlusion. Quickly and lightly massage the closed, affected eye and increas the patient's CO_2 level by using a mask or paper bag. A patient with retina detachment will present with sudden onset of seeing spots, lighting flashes, o sparks. Keep the patient's head immobilized. Both of these conditions requir immediate physician assessment.

In patients over 50 who have nausea and vomiting and ocular symptom consider closed-angle glaucoma.

ASSESSMENT

I. Initial observation
   A. Appearance of the eye: redness, tearing
   B. Ability to see
II. Subjective assessment
   A. History of onset and duration of symptoms
   B. Other related symptoms: headache, photophobia, nausea, and vomiting
   C. Alteration in vision: blurred, cloudy, loss of vision
   D. Pain
   E. Pertinent eye history
      1. Previous eye disorders
      2. Use of contact lenses or glasses
      3. History of eye injury in recent past, such as foreign body or abrasion
   F. Pertinent medical history
      1. Family history of eye problems (retinal detachments can be hereditary)

2. History of diabetes, hypertension, glaucoma
3. Medications and allergies

[I]I. Objective assessment

A. Physical assessment
1. Presence or absence of discharge from eye
2. Redness or edema
3. Presence of ulceration on the eyelid
4. Presence of abscesses along lid edges
5. Presence of lesions on cornea
6. Ocular mobility
7. Pupil equality, shape, and reactivity
8. Presence of pus or blood in anterior chamber

B. Visual acuity
1. Ability to discern light and shapes
2. Snellen chart test for each eye individually

C. Vital signs—any abnormalities, particularly in temperature and blood pressure, should be noted

OSSIBLE NURSING DIAGNOSES/ANALYSIS

I. Anxiety
I. Comfort, alteration in: pain
I. Coping, ineffective individual
V. Fear
V. Mobility, impaired physical
I. Sensory-perceptual alteration: visual

LANNING

. Priorities for care
A. Prevention of further damage
B. Pain control
C. Relief of anxiety

. Differential management

Condition	Clinical Assessment	Management
ACUTE ONSET OF BLINDNESS OR VISUAL FIELD REDUCTION WITHOUT TRAUMA		
Central Retinal Artery Occlusion	No history of trauma, sudden painless loss of vision; dilated nonreactive pupil	Lightly massage closed eye externally to decrease intraocular pressure; increase CO_2 level via rebreathing mask or paper bag; keep head of bed elevated; decrease intraocular pressure by having patient avoid coughing, sneezing, or bending over; obtain intravenous access; may be ordered to administer acetazolamide IV, mannitol IV, or timolol, one drop in affected eye, and nitroglycerin sublingually; ophthalmology consult
Acute Closed-Angle Glaucoma	Decreased visual acuity, nausea and vomiting; sudden, severe pain starting in one eye and radiating to head, blurred vision; patient may see halo around lights	Consult ophthalmology; obtain IV access; decrease intraocular pressure (as described above); relieve pain with analgesics; keep side rails up
Retinal Detachment	Alteration of vision; absence of pain; cloudy vision; seeing flashes or floaters	Keep patient's head immobilized; use bilateral eye patches; administer sedatives as ordered; keep side rails up; ophthalmology consult; surgical intervention
INFECTIONS		
Acute Conjunctivitis	Pink or red eye with variable discomfort, discharge; if viral: scant, watery drainage; if bacterial: thick and purulent discharge, clear cornea, equal pupils with normal light reaction, lid edema	Administer topical vasoconstrictors and antibiotics according to organism found

ndition	Clinical Assessment	Management
ratitis		
ctinic	(Refer to Chapter 31, Care Plan for Eye Injuries)	
ontact Lens	Caused by overuse of hard contact lens; eye pain bilaterally, blepharospasm, tearing	Remove contact lens; give short-acting cycloplegic; apply antibiotic ointment; patch both eyes
ute Iritis	Acute, moderately severe, unilateral pain; vision is blurred and patient is photophobic with small irregular pupils and lid edema	Administer 1% homatropine until patient is seen by ophthalmologist; apply warm compresses; give analgesics
rneal Ulcer		
Bacterial	Develops 1 to 2 days after corneal abrasion; painful red eye with diminished visual acuity	Immediate ophthalmology consult
Viral	Exclusively caused by herpes simplex; abrupt onset of discomfort, photophobia, tearing	Usually no treatment is needed; avoid use of steroids; patient should avoid known precipitants
ordeolum	Sty with pain and swelling	Apply warm compresses; give q.i.d. antibiotic ointment
epharitis	Irritated red eye; burning and itching; small ulcers on lids	Administer cleansing, compresses, antibiotic ointment

IPLEMENTATION

. Primary intervention
   A. Check visual acuity
      1. Check patient's eyes individually with a Snellen chart
      2. Physician may need to anesthetize eye
   B. Place patient supine or in semi-Fowler's position at rest; decrease lighting for patient's comfort
   C. Apply a sterile dressing or patch eyes as indicated
   D. Put side rails up; many patients have distorted depth perception
   E. Follow guidelines in differential section for specific eye problem

II. Secondary intervention
   A. Physician usually examines and treats patient; may need assistance
      retract eyelids, etc.
      1. Perform tonometry for suspected increased or decreased ocul
         pressure
      2. Instill drops: anesthetic, mydriatics, cycloplegics, or antibiotic
      3. Evaluate integrity of internal structures
      4. Administer parenteral analgesia or sedation as ordered
      5. Obtain cultures of purulent drainage if indicated
   B. Ophthalmology consult

EVALUATION

I. Patient outcomes/criteria
   A. Improvement in vision or no further deterioration
   B. Relief of anxiety
   C. Relief of pain
II. Document initial assessment data, emergency department interventio
    and patient's response to treatment
III. If previous patient outcomes are not reached, the emergency nurse shoul
     reevaluate the interventions and change the plan of care accordingly

DISPOSITION

I. Admission
   A. Acute glaucoma
   B. Retinal detachment
   C. Purulent conjunctivitis (gonorrhea)
   D. Retinal artery thrombosis
II. Discharge instructions
   A. Instructions
      1. Explain about eye condition according to diagnosis
      2. Discuss physician's instructions regarding activity and follow-up
      3. Warn patient of loss of depth perception with eye patch
   B. Follow-up
      1. Arrange appointment with ophthalmologist as indicated

CHAPTER 11

GASTROINTESTINAL BLEEDING

PLICATIONS FOR ACTION

e primary concern for emergency care in the patient with gastrointestinal I) bleeding is hemodynamic stabilization. It may not be possible to isolate e source of bleeding. The patient who arrives in the emergency department tively bleeding requires immediate attention directed toward volume resus-ation until he or she is hemodynamically stable. Implementation of the st-line plan is carried out before obtaining a thorough history and physical sessment.

SESSMENT

. Initial observation
   A. Skin color
   B. Level of consciousness
   C. Presence of blood or coffee ground emesis on face or clothes

. Subjective assessment
   A. History of blood in emesis or stool
      1. Color
      2. Amount
      3. Frequency
   B. Hematemesis generally indicates bleeding from stomach or proximal duodenum
   C. Melena
      1. May occur with or without hematemesis
      2. Usually requires at least 60 ml of blood and 6 to 8 hours in gastro-intestinal (GI) tract; if less time is involved, stool will appear ma-roon or bright red
      3. After cessation of bleeding, melena may persist for 48 to 72 hours; hemoccult positive stools may persist for 7 to 10 days

D. Associated symptoms
   1. Abdominal pain
   2. Weakness, fatigue
   3. Syncope
   4. Diarrhea
   5. Dyspnea
   6. Restlessness or anxiety

E. Significant history
   1. History of gastrointestinal bleeding, ulcer, or colon disease; coag lopathies; esophageal varices
   2. Medications: especially aspirin, anticoagulants, iron, antacids, st roids, antiinflammatory drugs
   3. Alcohol intake
   4. Caustic ingestion
   5. Consider swallowing of blood from epistaxis or oropharynge trauma as cause for hemoccult positive stool, hematemesis, coffee-ground emesis

III. Objective assessment

A. Orthostatic vital signs should be obtained if the patient is not tachyca dic at rest or when supine

B. Mental status
   1. Level of consciousness
   2. Orientation/appropriate behavior or conversation

C. Presence of petechiae, purpura, ecchymoses

D. Skin color: pale or jaundiced

E. Skin temperature, diaphoresis

F. Splenomegaly, liver enlargement

G. Bowel sounds
   1. Upper gastrointestinal bleeding: usually hyperactive
   2. Lower gastrointestinal bleeding: usually normal or hypoactive

POSSIBLE NURSING DIAGNOSES/ANALYSIS

I. Anxiety

II. Bowel elimination, alteration in:

III. Cardiac output, alteration in: decreased

IV. Comfort, alteration in: pain

V. Fluid volume deficit, actual or potential

VI. Knowledge deficit (of present illness)

VII. Noncompliance

VIII. Nutrition, alteration in: less than body requirements

IX. Tissue perfusion, alteration in: cerebral, cardiopulmonary, gastrointest nal, peripheral

ANNING

Priorities for care

A. Hemodynamic stabilization

B. Isolation of source of gastrointestinal bleeding

C. Gastric lavage for upper gastrointestinal bleeding

D. Airway management

Differential management

ndition	Clinical Assessment	Management
PPER GI BLEEDING		
astritis	Often associated with alcohol abuse, prolonged use of aspirin, antiinflammatory agents, iron, steroids, possibly spicy foods; epigastric pain, nausea and vomiting, anorexia; NG aspirate reveals fresh blood or coffee-ground material	Initiate IV hydration if patient is orthostatic or if vomiting persists, nasogastric (NG) lavage until clear of blood; give antacids, possibly antiemetics and antispasmodics; recommend patient avoid precipitating cause when possible
eptic Ulcer Disease astric and uodenal Ulcer)	Upper abdominal pain; food may bring relief or cause pain; history of documented ulcer disease or use of antacids is common; relief of pain may occur after a bleeding episode as blood acts as a buffer to gastric acid; tachycardia, hypotension if significant bleeding has occurred; NG aspirate reveals fresh blood or coffee-ground material	Initiate IV hydration, NG lavage until clear of blood; recommend patient avoid stimulants of acid production (caffeine, alcohol); give antacid therapy; surgery may be required if ulcer perforates
sophageal Varices	Caused by portal hypertension, tachycardia, hypotension; usually without pain; NG aspirate is grossly bloody and often prodigious	Initiate IV hydration; possible use of Sengstaken-Blakemore tube to apply controlled pressure against esophageal wall; administer vasopressin (Pitressin); surgical procedures may be needed (ligation, portacaval shunts)

Condition	Clinical Assessment	Management
Mallory-Weiss Syndrome	Tears in mucosal tissue of esophagus or stomach; multiple episodes of clear emesis followed by hematemesis, usually pain free	Initiate IV hydration; bleeding usually stops without specific treatmen although surgery may be necessary in some cases
LOWER GI BLEEDING		
Diverticulosis	Herniation of mucosa into muscle layer, which becomes inflamed; it is uncommon for patient to have diverticulitis and its complications concomitant with bleeding, hemorrhage; bleeding occurs from granulated tissue or erosion into blood vessel; patient has history of intermittent diarrhea, abdominal pain, flatulence	Initiate IV hydration; give liquid diet, stool softeners, and antibiotic therapy; barium enema may be therapeutic as well as diagnostic; surger sometimes necessary to control bleeding
Inflammatory (Ulcerative Colitis, Crohn's Disease)	Ulceration of mucosa; patient has abdominal pain, mild to severe bloody diarrhea, nausea and vomiting, fever with abscess and fistula formation	Initiate IV hydration; administer diet therapy, chronic drug therapy (corticosteroids, antidiarrheals)
Carcinoma	Changes in bowel patterns (diarrhea or constipation); bleeding may be occult; anorexia and weight loss, anemia, abdominal pain, distention	Admit for workup and surgical removal
Polyps	Growth from bowel wall, usually asymptomatic until bleeding occurs; patient may possibly have diarrhea and mucosal discharge	Initiate IV hydration; admit for workup; usually surgically removed

ndition	Clinical Assessment	Management
morrhoids	Varicosities of hemorrhoidal veins; may be internal or external to anal orifice; may bleed massively after surgical removal of clot in an internal hemorrhoid mistaken for a thrombosed external hemorrhoid; internal hemorrhoids more commonly bleed, usually painless	Apply moist heat; give stool softeners, local anesthetics; bed rest

PLEMENTATION

Primary intervention

A. Hemodynamic stabilization
   1. Establish intravenous access
      a) Use two large-bore peripheral IVs if patient is tachycardic or hypotensive; otherwise a single line is adequate
      b) Use CVP line if patient remains hypotensive
      c) Infuse normal saline or lactated Ringer's solution rapidly until patient is no longer hypotensive
   2. Place patient in Trendelenburg position; use pneumatic antishock trousers

B. Administer oxygen
   1. Intubate if patient is unresponsive and unable to maintain airway
   2. Give oxygen 4 to 8 L/min by mask or prongs if patient is hypotensive or anemic

C. Use cardiac monitor
   1. If patient tachycardic
   2. Other dysrhythmias are rare unless patient is severely anemic or hypotensive or has concomitant coronary artery disease; however, acute myocardial infarction (MI) can be precipitated by a hypotensive episode of gastrointestinal bleeding

D. Insert nasogastric tube
   1. Aspirate gastric contents to establish presence of blood; identify upper versus lower gastrointestinal bleeding

2. Perform gastric lavage
   - *a*) Use large-bore tube (Ewald 28 to 36) for acute bleeding
   - *b*) Administer lavage fluid: room temperature normal saline
   - *c*) Instill 200 to 300 ml of fluid and withdraw
   - *d*) Continue lavage until aspirate is clear of blood

E. Obtain laboratory data
1. Hematocrit
   - *a*) May be normal in massive, acute bleeding if equilibrium has n occurred
   - *b*) Low hematocrit usually indicates chronic bleeding
2. Hematest emesis and stool
3. Blood should be typed and held if patient is stable; type ar crossmatch 2 to 6 units for transfusion if patient is hypotensive tachycardic; packed cells for chronic bleeding
4. PT/PTT, platelet count
5. Electrolytes, glucose
6. Liver function tests

F. Transfuse blood products and fresh frozen plasma as ordered; vitamin administration as indicated

II. Secondary intervention

A. Take serial vital signs; repeat hematocrit after IV hydration

B. Insert indwelling urinary catheter if patient is in shock

C. Administer medications
1. Antacids
   - *a*) Maalox: 30 to 60 ml orally or by nasogastric tube when bleedir has ceased
   - *b*) Cimetidine
     - (1) Histamine antagonist
     - (2) 300 mg IV; also available in oral dose
2. Vasopressin (Pitressin)
   - *a*) Indicated for upper gastrointestinal bleeding caused by esop ageal varices
   - *b*) 20 units IV over 10 minutes; then 0.2 to 0.6 units/min; taper do slowly, never stop abruptly
   - *c*) Contraindicated in patients with coronary artery disease as may precipitate an acute myocardial infarction

3. Vitamin K (AquaMEPHYTON)
    a) Treatment for Coumadin toxicity
    b) 10 to 40 mg IV
4. Oral antibiotic (neomycin) or lactolose
    a) Indicated for prevention of hepatic encephalopathy
    b) Prevents protein breakdown of blood in gastrointestinal tract to reduce ammonia production

D. Provide emotional support to patient and family
E. Arrange for medicine or surgical consultation as indicated

VALUATION

I. Patient outcomes/criteria
  A. Bleeding controlled; source identified if possible
  B. Vital signs within normal limits
  C. Appropriate mental status

I. Document initial assessment data, emergency department intervention, and patient's response to treatment

I. If previous patient outcomes are not reached, the emergency nurse should reevaluate the interventions and change the plan of care accordingly

ISPOSITION

Admission criteria
  A. Hemodynamically unstable
  B. Unable to control bleeding or isolate source
  C. Abnormal clotting studies

Discharge guidelines
  A. Arrange outpatient workup for GI series, endoscopy, when appropriate
  B. Recommend patient avoid precipitating factors (alcohol, caffeine, stress, dietary factors)
  C. Give medications
    1. Antacids
    2. Cimetidine
    3. Sucraflate (coats mucosal defects)
  D. Instruct patient to return if symptoms recur

CHAPTER 12

HEADACHE

IMPLICATIONS FOR ACTION

The large majority of patients who come to the emergency department w headache are considered to be stable since most are only disabled by the pa A small percentage, however, are true emergencies. The emergency nu must treat each patient presenting with a headache as a true emergency ur proven otherwise. Early red flags that will alert the nurse are sudden onset severe or unusual headache, progression, recent change in duration and f quency, presence of lethargy or decreased mentation, history of recent a remote head trauma, diastolic blood pressure of 130 mm Hg or greater, pr ence of nuchal rigidity or any motor deficits. If patient complains of "wo headache ever experienced" this should trigger concern. If any of these a present, the nurse should proceed to the implementation section of the ca plan. Those interventions should be carried out before obtaining a thorou history and physical assessment.

ASSESSMENT

I. Initial observation
   A. Level of consciousness
   B. Appearance indicative of pain
II. Subjective assessment
   A. Description of event
      1. Onset and duration of pain
      2. Character: sharp, dull, throbbing
      3. Location
      4. Intensity, compared to previous headaches
      5. Mode of onset: presence or absence of prodromal symptoms, fla ing lights, blurry vision, foods, menses, etc.
   B. Associated symptoms
      1. Nausea and vomiting
      2. Blurry vision or photophobia
      3. Dizziness or vertigo

4. Behavioral changes
5. Drowsiness, confusion
6. Paresthesia
7. Fever or chills

C. Past medical history
1. History of recurrent headaches
a) Diagnosis, if known
b) Frequency
c) Usual treatment
2. Recent or remote head trauma
3. Medications and allergies
4. Chronic diseases

I. Objective assessment
A. Vital signs—especially temperature and blood pressure
B. Neurological status
1. Use Glasgow coma scale
2. Motor strength
C. Signs of trauma
1. Ecchymosis
2. Hematoma
3. Lacerations, abrasions

OSSIBLE NURSING DIAGNOSES/ANALYSIS

I. Anxiety
I. Comfort, alteration in: pain
I. Tissue perfusion, alteration in: cerebral
V. Sensory-perceptual alteration: visual, tactile, olfactory
V. Any nursing diagnosis that might be a cause of stress for the patient
A. Sleep pattern disturbance
B. Social isolation
C. Spiritual distress (distress of the human spirit)

LANNING

Priorities for care
A. Prepare for emergency procedures in patient with rapidly decreasing neurological status
1. Assure airway, breathing, and circulation (ABCs)
2. Maintain blood pressure control
3. Attempt to prevent or treat seizures
B. Decrease environmental stimuli
C. Decrease anxiety by providing reassurance and emotional support

Differential management

Type	Clinical Assessment	Management
TENSION		
	Caused by muscular contractions; gradual onset; bandlike pressure; often psychosocial factors involved	Administer mild analgesi[cs], mild tranquilizers, nonsteroidal anti-inflammatory agents
VASCULAR		
	(Caused by vasodilatation after a variable period of vasoconstriction)	
Migraine	Usually throbbing, unilateral, and associated with nausea, vomiting, photophobia; more common in women; often patients have prodromal symptoms before onset of pain; often psychosocial factors are involved	Administer ergotamine tartrate (Cafergot), propranolol; patient may also receive narcotic or sedative
Cluster	Frequent headaches in short periods of time, unilateral; without prodrome or nausea or vomiting; more common in middle-aged male smokers; due to autonomic disorder	Administer propranolol, lithium carbonate, steroids, ergotamine tartrate (Cafergot), or methysergide maleate
Hypertension (NOTE: Does not usually cause headache unless diastolic pressure is sustained above 130 mm Hg)	Pounding or throbbing, usually occipital region; headache is the most consistent symptom related directly to elevated blood pressure; usually worse in the morning, generally improves during the day	
	Four categories of headaches:	
	1. Recent onset of persistent headache unrelated to hypertension	Give analgesia

ndition	Clinical Assessment	Management
	2. Significant hypertension on arrival in emergency department with global, throbbing headache	Maintain blood pressure control; give analgesia
	3. Hypertensive crisis with change in mentation; headache followed by mental changes, blurred vision, aphasia, seizures	Obtain IV access, maintain blood pressure control; give analgesia; admit for observation; if nitroprusside lowers blood pressure and mentation returns, then crisis can be differentiated from cerebral vascular accident
	4. Pheochromocytoma—patient will have increased hypertension, headache, nausea, vomiting, sweating, flushes of face, palpitations	Manage blood pressure with alpha- and beta-blocking agents and with nitroprusside as necessary
her Vascular adaches (postictal tes; acute mountain kness; histamine headaes; nitrite and nitrate adaches; "hangovers"; adaches caused by poglycemia, marijuana, rebound from caffeine)	History very important in making diagnosis	Withdrawal from precipitating factor
UG WITHDRAWAL OR INTERACTION		
	Headache caused by withdrawal from clonidine or propranolol or interaction of MAO inhibitors and Chianti wine	Treat underlying cause

Condition	Clinical Assessment	Management
TRACTION (CAUSED BY PRESSURE ON PAIN-SENSITIVE STRUCTURES)		
Bleeding		
Subarachnoid hemorrhage	Severe, abrupt onset; patient may have nausea, vomiting, or low grade fever; nuchal rigidity; often caused by leaking arterial aneurysm; lumbar puncture reveals bloody cerebrospinal fluid (CSF); may also be caused by trauma	CT scan; surgical interv tion; may require blo pressure control
Epidural	Follows trauma; patient may or may not recall trauma; usually caused by arterial blood associated with skull fracture; patient may be awake and alert and then rapidly lose consciousness	CT scan; surgical intervention
Subdural	Follows trauma; may be acute or chronic, often found in alcoholics; (NOTE: patient may not remember trauma)	CT scan; surgical intervention
Cerebral vascular accident and intracerebral bleeding	Main cause is hypertension; can be caused by trauma; often focal findings more prominent than headache; most often secondary to thrombosis	CT scan; surgical intervention
Tumors	Headache moderate, intermittent; usually there are focal findings and abnormal mental status	CT scan; surgical intervention
Abscess	Headache similar to that of tumor headache	Administer antibiotics; surgical intervention

ndition	Clinical Assessment	Management
FLAMMATION		
eningitis	Diffuse headache accompanied by fever, nuchal rigidity, pain with ocular motion	Assist in lumbar puncture with cell count and gram stain 1. Bacterial origin: treated with antibiotics specific to causal organism 2. Viral origin: may not require admission, only rest and mild analgesia
mporal Arteritis	Occurs usually in patients over 50, mild headache; can be accompanied by intense visual dimming; low grade fever, muscle pain, joint pain; usually unilateral, prominent in area of temporal arteries	Obtain sedimentation rate, complete blood count; CT scan; assist with lumbar puncture; give steroids and analgesia
igeminal Neuralgia	Stabbing severe pain distributed along trigeminal nerve; usually unilateral; facial movement or palpation increases pain	Administer parenteral analgesia, carbamazepine
us Headache	Patient may have fever, irritability, malaise, disturbed sense of smell, tenderness to palpation over involved sinus, purulent nasal discharge, constant dull aching, severe pain	Administer analgesia, antibiotics, and heat; recommend rest; admission and surgery for multiple sinus involvement
TRACRANIAL ORIGINS		
chogenic	Caused by depressed, delusional, conversional, or hypochondrial states; any type of manifestation; by history pain does not inconvenience patient (such as no interference with work, sleep, or play)	No neurological pathology; recommend psychotherapy

Condition	Clinical Assessment	Management
Glaucoma	Intense orbital and periorbital pain with acute onset; patient may have nausea or vomiting; visual haziness or loss; possible conjunctivitis and lid congestion	Measure intraocular pre sure; administer appropriate medication
POST–HEAD INJURY		
	May persist for days; often accompanied by nausea, vomiting, and vertigo	Administer mild analges have patient lie flat, which usually brings relief

IMPLEMENTATION

I. Primary intervention
   A. Manage airway
      1. If ventilations are inadequate, oxygenate patient with ambu-b mask, and prepare to intubate
      2. If ventilations are adequate, administer oxygen 3 to 6 L/min via na prongs
   B. Obtain intravenous access
      1. For severe or unusual headache
      2. Any change in level of consciousness
      3. Diastolic blood pressure of 140 mm Hg or greater
      4. For infusion of dextrose 5% with microdrip at a TKO rate
   C. Follow guidelines in differential management section according to s cific etiology of headache
   D. Control seizures (Refer to Chapter 23, Care Plan for Seizures)
   E. Administer medications
      1. Nitroprusside
         a) 50 mg vial in 250, 500, or 1000 ml dextrose 5% solution; inf at 0.5 to 10 μg/kg/min; wrap bottle with aluminum foil
         b) Obtain baseline vital signs before starting infusion
         c) Check vital signs q5 min for first 30 min, then q15 min thereaf
         d) Discontinue drip for severe hypotension
         e) Run in peripheral IV with no other drug

2. Diazoxide
   a) Administer 300 mg IV push bolus in 30 seconds or less
   b) Monitor intake and output
   c) Advise patient to move cautiously by rising slowly or avoiding sudden position changes to minimize orthostatic hypotension
3. Apresoline: 20 to 40 mg IV slowly
4. Furosemide: 20 to 80 mg IV push over 2 to 4 minutes
5. Mannitol: 50 to 200 gm of 20% solution over 20 to 60 min IV
6. Analgesic medications according to physician preference
7. Ergotamine tartrate
8. Carbamazepine for trigeminal neuralgia: up to 1200 mg/day to achieve freedom from pain

F. Carefully monitor changes in level of consciousness
G. Decrease environmental stimuli
   1. Darken room
   2. Decrease noise
   3. Limit visitors
H. Obtain laboratory data as outlined in differential management section

. Secondary intervention
   A. Prepare for procedures outlined in differential management section according to specific etiology
   B. Provide emotional support and reassurance

VALUATION

I. Patient outcomes/criteria
   A. Level of consciousness remains stable or does not deteriorate
   B. Vital signs within normal range
   C. Relief or diminution of pain

I. Document initial assessment data, emergency department intervention, and patient's response to treatment

I. If previous patient outcomes are not reached, the emergency nurse should reevaluate the interventions and change the plan of care accordingly

DISPOSITION

I. Admission criteria
   A. Conditions that require treatment or observation unable to be impl mented at home (i.e., IV, antibiotics)

II. Discharge guidelines
   A. Explain head injury instructions where appropriate to patient and i structions to return for increase in pain, vomiting, or change in me tation
   B. Encourage compliance with follow-up examination at physician's offic
   C. Refer patient for nonpharmacological treatment (if needed), such biofeedback, transcutaneous nerve stimulation, psychotherapy, relax tion therapy, or exercise programs

CHAPTER 13

HEMOPHILIA

MPLICATIONS FOR ACTION

The majority of patients entering the emergency department with a hemophilia-related problem have been previously diagnosed with the disorder. The most frequent presentation is soft tissue or joint bleeding as a result of minor trauma. Immediate and adequate factor replacement is the primary goal along with assessment of patient and family educational needs.

ASSESSMENT

I. Initial observation
   A. Obvious external bleeding
   B. Posture indicative of pain
   C. Level of consciousness
II. Subject assessment
   A. History of hemophilia
   B. Time and location symptoms began; tingling or pain is usually the first symptom to indicate bleeding
   C. Recent trauma
   D. Associated history or symptoms
      1. Syncope: possible blood loss or intracranial bleeding
      2. Headache, nausea and vomiting, blurry vision, recent seizure activity or changes in mental status: consider intracranial hemorrhage
      3. Sore throat may indicate retropharyngeal bleeding
      4. Abdominal pain, hematemesis, or melena: indicative of gastrointestinal bleeding
      5. Back pain may be symptom of retroperitoneal bleeding or renal bleeding
II. Objective assessment
   A. Vital signs
      1. Tachycardia often present
      2. Obtain orthostatic vital signs, if not hypotensive
      3. Fever may accompany joint hemorrhage

B. Skin color
   1. Pallor may be related to vasoconstriction as a compensatory mec anism of significant bleeding
   2. Ecchymosis; subcutaneous hematoma may be present without (chymosis
C. Skin may feel warm over bleeding site
D. Most common sites of joint bleeding are elbows, knees, and ankl• patient may be unable to walk or use affected joints
E. Neurological assessment should be obtained; altered mental status m indicate intracranial hemorrhage, which is the leading cause of death persons with hemophilia (25% to 30%)
F. Neurovascular assessment of extremity if there is joint or soft tiss• bleeding; consider measuring circumferences to compare sides

POSSIBLE NURSING DIAGNOSES/ANALYSIS

I. Activity intolerance
II. Anxiety
III. Comfort, alteration in: pain
IV. Coping, ineffective individual and family: compromised
V. Fluid volume deficit, actual and potential
VI. Home maintenance management, impaired
VII. Injury: potential for trauma
VIII. Knowledge deficit (of disease process of hemophilia)
IX. Self-concept, disturbance in: body image and personal identity
X. Skin integrity, impairment of: actual
XI. Tissue perfusion, alteration in: peripheral

PLANNING

I. Priorities for care
   A. Treat hypovolemia
   B. Undertake factor replacement
   C. Isolate source of bleeding
   D. Administer analgesia
II. Pathophysiology
   A. Hemophilia A (classic)
      1. X-linked recessive trait, therefore clinically evident in males; femal• are carriers
      2. Decreased functional level of factor VIII
   B. Hemophilia B (Christmas disease)
      1. Same genetics as hemophilia A
      2. Decreased functional level of factor IX

C. Classification
   1. Mild
      a) Factors VIII and IX: 5% to 25% (% present)
      b) Bleeding occurs as a result of trauma or surgery
   2. Moderate
      a) Factors VIII and IX: 2% to 5% (% present)
      b) Bleeding occurs as a result of mild trauma, at times spontaneously
   3. Severe
      a) Factors VIII and IX: 0% to 1% (% present)
      b) Patient may have frequent, spontaneous bleeding

D. von Willebrand's disease
   1. Hemorrhagic syndrome caused by deficiencies of a molecule on the factor VIII complex
   2. Involves ecchymosis and bleeding of mucous membranes

E. Laboratory findings in different hemophilias
   1. Significant bleeding results in decreased hematocrit
   2. Normal protime (PT)
   3. Normal platelet count
   4. Prolonged partial thromboplastin time (PTT)
   5. Bleeding time normal in hemophilia A and B; prolonged in von Willebrand's disease

IPLEMENTATION

Primary intervention

A. Provide intravenous access for hydration and factor replacement

B. Obtain hematocrit; type and crossmatch for massive, acute bleeding

C. Determine types of factor replacement
   1. Factor VIII concentrate
      a) Treatment for hemophilia A
      b) Obtained by purification of cryoprecipitate, therefore less volume infused
      c) Adult and pediatric dose: number of units required = 0.5 wt (kg) × desired increment % of factor VIII level
      d) Vials are usually 280 to 300 units/vial
   2. Cryoprecipitate
      a) Made from thawing fresh frozen plasma and collecting precipitate
      b) High in fibrinogen
      c) One bag cryoprecipitate equivalent to approximately 100 units of factor VIII

- *d*) Recommended units are same as factor VIII concentrate
- *e*) Thaw in 37-degree C bath for 5 to 10 minutes; higher heat v destroy protein
- *f*) Withdraw cryoprecipitate from bag using Y-type blood com nent set with filter
- *g*) Administer cryoprecipitate IV push through the filter over proximately 5 minutes
- *h*) Do not use cryoprecipitate if it appears clumped or clotted

3. Factor IX
   - *a*) Treatment for patients with hemophilia A with inhibitor hemophilia B
   - *b*) Activates factor IX without relying on factor VIII
   - *c*) Hemolysis can occur with high doses or prolonged treatmen
   - *d*) Recommended dose for hemophilia A with inhibitor: 50 to units/kg
   - *e*) Recommended dose for hemophilia B: number of units requir = 1 × wt (kg) × desired % increment
   - *f*) Autoplex or antiinhibitor complex is used in hemophilia A wit high titer of inhibitor or with serious bleeding
4. Fresh frozen plasma
   - *a*) Used in treatment of hemophilia A or B
   - *b*) Use caution to avoid volume overload
   - *c*) 1 ml is equivalent to approximately 1 unit of factor VIII or I
5. Whole blood is used only in massive, acute bleeding to restore blo volume
6. Aminocaproic acid (Amicar)
   - *a*) Inhibitor of fibrinolytic enzymes
   - *b*) Treatment for bleeding or oral mucosa during dental procedur
   - *c*) Usually given in conjunction with factor replacement
   - *d*) Patients should avoid placing glass, metal, or sharp objects mouth
   - *e*) Liquid or soft diet for 24 to 48 hours

D. Transfusion or allergic reaction to factor replacement may occur shor after administration
   1. Indicated by hives, rash, uticaria, flushing, wheezing
   2. Treat with Benadryl

E. Patients with suspected intracranial pathology will need CT scan

F. Pressure at needle site should be held for 5 minutes after intraveno line is discontinued

G. Bleeding joints should be immobilized in extended position; apply ice bag if bleeding is recent or continued

Secondary intervention

A. Observe for compartment syndrome in soft tissue bleeding
B. Give analgesia
   1. Pain may diminish soon after bleeding ceases
   2. Avoid aspirin or other medications that have antiplatelet function
   3. Appropriate medications include acetaminophen, propoxyphene, pentazocine, codeine, morphine, meperidine, dihydromorphinone
   4. Antiinflammatory agents are used to treat degenerative joint disease
C. Consider associated illness
   1. Hepatitis: obtain liver enzymes
   2. Acquired Immune Deficiency Syndrome (AIDS)
   3. Drug dependency
   4. Urinalysis to detect hematuria
   5. Degenerative joint disease
D. Support patient and family
   1. Assess learning needs surrounding disease and therapy
   2. Evaluate home maintenance and follow-up care
   3. Refer with careful follow-up to appropriate hematologist; patient must be encouraged not to bounce from emergency department to emergency department and he or she should know what factor is needed
   4. Provide good med-alert identification

VALUATION

I. Patient outcomes/criteria
   A. Vital signs within normal limits
   B. Hemostasis
   C. Normal mental status
   D. Relief of pain
I. Document initial assessment, emergency department intervention, and patient's response to treatment
I. If previous patient outcomes are not reached, the emergency nurse should reevaluate the interventions and change the plan of care accordingly

DISPOSITION

I. Admission criteria
   A. Head trauma, CNS bleeding
   B. Persistent headache
   C. Acute internal bleeding, such as gastrointestinal bleeding or retr peritoneal bleeding
   D. Unstable vital signs
   E. Persistent bleeding that does not respond to factor replacement
   F. Pharyngeal bleeding
   G. Soft tissue bleeding with compartment syndrome
   H. Progressive joint bleeding

II. Discharge guidelines
   A. Provide appropriate hematology consult for follow-up care
   B. Consider telephone consult 24 to 48 hours after factor replacement
   C. If patient is involved in home therapy, assess availability of factor
   D. Ensure patient and family have clear understanding of when and whe to seek emergency care

CHAPTER 14

HYPERTHERMIA

IPLICATIONS FOR ACTION

yperthermia involves a spectrum of diseases as the body tries to maintain a ormal temperature when it encounters a large environmental or internal heat ad. Most individuals who seek medical treatment have heat disorders that are e result of environmental temperature of 90 degrees F (30 degrees C) or ove. In those situations where the cause is clearly environmental, the emerncy nurse can quickly take the patient's rectal temperature and assess hether the patient is experiencing a heat exhaustion temperature of 37.8 grees C (100 degrees F) or a heatstroke temperature above 40.5 degrees C 05 degrees F). If the patient's temperature exceeds 38 degrees and the cause a probable heatstroke, start aggressive cooling measures immediately (see nplementation section). Do not wait to draw blood or assess patient further heatstroke may be rapidly fatal.

SSESSMENT

I. Initial observation
  A. Respiratory status
  B. Skin: color and moisture
  C. Level of consciousness
II. Subjective assessment
  A. History of hyperthermic episode
    1. High humidity (humid outdoor environment, sauna, or hot tubs)
    2. High heat (summertime heat or heavy clothing)
    3. Cause of exposure such as alcohol or drugs, dementia, or injury
    4. Strenuous exercise (athletes, soldiers most susceptible)
  B. Pertinent medical history
    1. Current febrile condition
    2. Previous heat illness
    3. Chronic disease (diabetes, seizures, obesity, malnutrition, scleroderma, cystic fibrosis)

4. Medication
   a) Drugs that increase heat production (amphetamines, barbit rates, LSD)
   b) Drugs that decrease heat dissipation (phenothiazines, antich linergics, diuretics, propranolol)
5. Allergies

C. Age-at-risk groups
   1. Elderly
   2. Neonates

D. Associated symptoms
   1. Gastrointestinal upset: anorexia, nausea, vomiting
   2. Central nervous system (CNS) dysfunction: headache, dizzines syncope, irritability, confusion, coma
   3. Pain
      a) Heat cramps—associated with muscles that have been exte sively used, such as calf muscles
      b) Chest pain

III. Objective assessment
   A. Complete vital signs
      1. Rectal temperature
      2. Orthostatic blood pressure changes may occur with heat exhau tion
      3. Tachycardia
   B. Respiratory status—can vary from normal to hyperventilation or hyp ventilation
   C. Level of consciousness—will vary from irritability to frank coma; se zures may occur
   D. Skin—can vary from hot, flushed, and diaphoretic with heat exhaustio to anhidrotic skin with heatstroke
   E. Muscle twitching
   F. Oliguria

POSSIBLE NURSING DIAGNOSES/ANALYSIS

I. Cardiac output, alteration in: decreased
II. Fluid volume deficit, actual
III. Knowledge deficit (of environmental heat hazards)
IV. Tissue perfusion, alteration in: cerebral, cardiopulmonary, renal, gastr intestinal, peripheral
V. Urinary elimination, alteration in patterns

ANNING

Priorities for care

A. Control and maintenance of airway, breathing, and circulation (ABCs)

B. Restoration and maintenance of normothermia, cooling patient rapidly

C. Hydration

D. Isolating cause of hyperthermia if not readily apparent

Differential management

ndition	Clinical Assessment	Management
AT EDEMA	Mild swelling of extremities; pitting edema of the ankles	No special treatment required
AT TETANY	Carpopedal spasms occurring during exposure to heat	Removal of patient to cool environment
AT SYNCOPE	Usually occurs in unacclimatized subjects during early stages of heat exposure; hypotension	Rest and removal from heat stress; avoidance of any quick movements or prolonged standing
ICKLY HEAT	Superficial glistening vesicles on a red base; itching; usually found on body parts that are clothed	Apply chlorhexidine lotion to affected areas; air-conditioned environment 8-12 hours daily helpful; if rash becomes diffuse and pustular, antibiotics may be considered
HIDROTIC HEAT	Usually preceded by prickly heat; excessive fatigue in response to physical exertion; failure of normal sweating; tachycardia and tachypnea; temperature to 38 degrees C	Have patient avoid exertion; cool environment; administer potassium supplements as indicated by electrolyte laboratory values

Condition	Clinical Assessment	Management
HEAT CRAMPS		
	Cramps of most worked muscles usually after exertion; no hyperventilation noted; patient may also complain of weakness, headache, and nausea	Give salt replacement orally or intravenously; rest in cool environment
HEAT EXHAUSTION		
(NOTE: Distinction from heatstroke is that mental function remains intact)	Headache, giddiness, anorexia, thirst, vomiting; temperature elevation to 40 degrees C, increased pulse, and increased respiratory rate; orthostatic blood pressure changes; anxiety and irritability	Provide cool environment; perform hydration—orally or intravenously based on laboratory findings; IV fluid choice dextrose 5%/0.45 sodium chloride
HEATSTROKE		
Non-exercise (occurs in elderly with cardiovascular disease, in obese persons with cardiovascular disease, and in people on thyroid compounds or amphetamines) **Exercise induced** (occurs in athletes, soldiers, laborers, or anyone who is unable to dissipate body heat after strenuous exercise)	Rectal temperature greater than 41 degrees C; altered level of consciousness; hot, dry skin; rapid respiration; tachycardia; hypotension; seizures; coma	Rapidly cool patient's body until temperature reaches 38.5 degrees C; intubate if comatose; provide IV access, fluid choice dextrose 5%/0.45 normal saline if hypotensive 0.9 normal saline; administer oxygen 5 to 10 L/min; continuously monitor rectal temperature; insert venous pressure line and indwelling urinary catheter (NOTE: Children experiencing hyperthermia may require same cooling treatment as adults)

IPLEMENTATION

Primary intervention

A. Cool body rapidly
   1. Cover naked patient with sheet that is wet with ice water and ice chips; give priority to axilla and groin
   2. Keep patient's skin wet with warm water and keep fan blowing on patient; discontinue when patient's temperature reaches 38.5 degrees C rectally
   3. Apply hypothermia blanket to thorax

B. Maintain airway—intubate if necessary; coma, seizures, and vomiting common in heatstroke; administration of oxygen 5 to 10 L/min via nasal prongs is helpful

C. Obtain intravenous access where appropriate; fluid choice dextrose 5%/0.45 normal saline; if hypotensive, 0.9 normal saline

D. Follow guidelines in differential management section

E. Cardiac monitoring: expect ST depression, T wave changes, bundle branch blocks, ventricular fibrillation
   1. Provide continuous bedside monitoring
   2. Obtain 12-lead ECG

F. Provide central venous pressure monitor and indwelling urinary catheter to assess volume and perfusion

Secondary intervention

A. Perform laboratory studies
   1. Baseline: complete blood count, electrolytes, BUN, creatine, glucose, PT/PTT, ABGs, SGOT, LDH, CPK; elevations of SGOT, LDH, and CPK will help differentiate heatstroke from heat exhaustion
   2. Others as indicated: alcohol and drug screen

B. Serially monitor
   1. Temperature via continuous rectal probe
   2. Fluid status—observe for any signs of pulmonary edema

C. Administer medications as indicated
   1. Isoproterenol or dopamine considered for shock, titrated to blood pressure readings
   2. Chlorpromazine: 25 to 50 mg IV to control shivering
   3. Diazepam: 5 to 10 mg IV for seizures
   4. Mannitol: 12.5 gm IV to promote renal blood flow
   5. Sodium bicarbonate to correct acidosis

D. Treat associated problems and injuries as indicated

E. Explain treatment to patient and family as needed

EVALUATION

I. Patient outcomes/criteria
   A. Return to normothermia
   B. Improved neurological status
   C. Lack of shivering during cooling
   D. Vital signs within normal limits
II. Document initial assessment data, emergency department interventio and patient's response to treatment
III. If previous patient outcomes are not reached, the emergency nurse shoul reevaluate the interventions and change the plan of care accordingly

DISPOSITION

I. Admission criteria
   A. Heatstroke may require admission for 24 hours of observation; may onl require admission to Emergency Medical Services observation unit fo fluid and electrolyte replacement
   B. Admit to intensive care if complications occur in emergency depart ment
II. Discharge guidelines
   A. Heat cramps and heat exhaustion can usually be managed in the emer gency department with cooling and replacement of salt and fluid de pletion
   B. Teach preventative measures to patient and family
      1. Decrease in exertional activity in hot humid weather
      2. Replacement of fluids and salt in hot weather
      3. Dressing in light and loose-fitting clothing
      4. Getting frequent rest and cooling during hot humid weather
      5. Acclimating to the climate slowly
   C. Refer to physician for follow-up if problems arise or there is continua tion of gastrointestinal disturbances such as anorexia, nausea, or vomit ing

HAPTER 15

HYPOTHERMIA

PLICATIONS FOR ACTION

ypothermia occurs when the body's core temperature drops below 35 de-ees C (95 degrees F). It usually occurs in patients who are exposed to cold cool, wet, and windy conditions. In most situations in which the exposure is vious, nursing actions will be straightforward. They include:

1. CPR if necessary (until patient is resuscitated successfully or is re-warmed to 32 degrees C, then declared dead)
2. Gentle handling to avoid precipitating ventricular fibrillation
3. Fluid replacement and rewarming

ose patients who come to the emergency department with subtle progres-n of hypothermia may demonstrate the following: fatigue and progressive athy or lack of cooperation; the elderly may have slow progression of mental terioration, mimicking senility; or some patients may have slurred speech d ataxia mimicking a cerebrovascular accident. Hypothermia can also be a gn of metabolic failure and can occur at normal or elevated environmental mperatures.

SSESSMENT

. Initial observation
   A. Level of consciousness
   B. Respiratory status
   C. Color of mucous membranes and extremities
   D. Skin temperature

I. Subjective assessment
   A. History of hypothermic episode
      1. Length of exposure and environment (in or out of doors)
      2. Presence of wind or water
      3. Cause of exposure, such as alcohol or drugs, dementia, debility, injury

B. Pertinent medical history
   1. Chronic or acute illness: causes of hypothermia include myxedem hypopituitarism, hypoglycemia, hypoadrenalism, Wernicke's sy drome, sepsis, or ingestion of drugs such as ethanol, barbiturate and phenothiazine
   2. Medication and allergies, immunization status
   3. Predisposing factors, such as age, infirmity, or economic hardship

III. Objective assessment
A. Complete vital signs
   1. Hypothermic patient often unrecognized until initial temperatu taken; hypothermia defined as 35 degrees C (95 degrees F) or belo
   2. Rectal temperature
      a) Rectal probe must be used if temperature is less than 34 degre C (93.2 F)
      b) Mild hypothermia: 32 to 35 degrees C (89.6 to 95 F)
      Moderate hypothermia: 30 to 32 degrees C (86 to 89.6 F)
      Severe hypothermia: less than 30 degrees C (86 F)
   3. Respiratory status: increased respiration in mild cases, decrease respirations in moderate, apnea in severe
   4. Presence of distal pulses

B. Level of consciousness
   1. Mild hypothermia (above 32 degrees C [89.6 F]): dulled mentatio generally oriented
   2. Moderate and severe hypothermia (below 32 degrees C [89.6 F] disorientation, confusion, lethargy, progressing to stupor or coma

C. Muscle activity
   1. Mild hypothermia (above 32 degrees C [89.6 F]): shivering, ur coordinated movements, staggering gait
   2. Severe and moderate hypothermia (below 32 degrees C [89.6 F] no shivering; patient unable to perform meaningful tasks; muscle may simulate rigor mortis in severe hypothermic stage

POSSIBLE NURSING DIAGNOSES/ANALYSIS

I. Breathing pattern, ineffective
II. Cardiac output, alteration in: decreased
III. Fluid volume deficit, actual
IV. Knowledge deficit (of environmental cold hazards)
V. Skin integrity, impairment of: actual
VI. Tissue perfusion, alteration in: cerebral, cardiopulmonary, peripheral

ANNING

Priorities for care

A. Control and maintenance of airway, breathing, and circulation (ABCs)

B. Restore and maintain normothermia

C. Prevent the development of complications during therapeutic procedures

Differential management

ndition	Clinical Assessment	Management
GREE OF HYPOTHERMIA		
ld (32-35° C .6-95° F])	Increased blood pressure, heart rate, respiratory rate; shivering, developing ataxia, diuresis	Passive external rewarming: blankets, warm room
oderate 0-32° C 6-89.6° F])	Decreased heart rate and respiratory rate; decreased clearing of secretions; decreased level of consciousness; fine tremors; decreased pain sensitivity; ventricular fibrillation susceptibility	Passive external rewarming; active internal and external rewarming; give warm intravenous fluids; provide heated oxygen mist, heated peritoneal dialysis, gastric or bladder lavage (NOTE: AVOID warming extremities during active rewarming to prevent rush of cold blood from periphery to core, which can cause core temperature afterdrop)
vere (<30° C 6° F])	Unresponsive, no shivering, dysrhythmias; no reflexes or response to pain; significant hypotension; maximum risk of ventricular fibrillation; rigor mortis–like state	Undertake measures for moderate hypothermia plus thoracotomy with mediastinal lavage with heated fluid; extracorporeal blood rewarming (heated hemodialysis); cardiovascular bypass for rapid core rewarming with advanced life support measures

Condition	Clinical Assessment	Management
FROSTBITE (MAY BE SEEN IN CONJUNCTION WITH HYPOTHERMIA OR BY ITSELF)		
Superficial	Skin whitish, does not blanch when pressed; pain is sharp or aching; patient may complain of some loss of feeling	Rapid rewarming of extremity immerse in warm bath 40.5 degrees C (105 F); handle gently; keep patient immersed until flushed warm to touch with blanching; place sterile cotton between digits; administer analgesia
Deep	Patient complains of numbness, heaviness, or complete loss of sensation; tissue: skin appears pale, waxy, remains cold, mottled blue or gray after rewarming	Same as for superficial hospitalization; treat as bad burn (refer to Chapter 39, Care Plan for Surface Trauma: Burns)

IMPLEMENTATION

I. Primary intervention
   A. If cardiopulmonary resuscitation is necessary, it must be continued unti temperature is above 32 degrees C (89.6 F); medication and defibrilla tion are not effective at lower temperatures
   B. Give 100% oxygen via heated nebulizer; intubation may stimulate ven tricular fibrillation, so if necessary, preoxygenate
   C. Insert large-bore IV—rapid infusion
      1. Warm dextrose 5% or dextrose 5% half normal saline; will depend on results of laboratory results; avoid lactated Ringer's since hypo thermic liver cannot metabolize lactate
      2. Dextrose 50% and naloxone for patient who is unresponsive
   D. Bedside cardiac monitoring
      1. Expect dysrhythmias, especially atrial fibrillation, premature ven tricular contractions, conduction blocks, ventricular fibrillation, Os borne or J wave
      2. Obtain 12-lead ECG
   E. Insert indwelling urinary catheter to assess volume and perfusion
   F. Manage temperature
      1. Remove all patient's clothing, particularly if wet
      2. Insert rectal probe for continuous monitoring

3. Begin rewarming methods; core rewarming must precede or accompany peripheral, as peripheral demands could exceed capacity of cold heart
    a) Passive external: for mild hypothermia only; cover patient with warm blankets and allow to rewarm
    b) Active external: cover patient with heated blankets or immerse in warm water (difficult to manage in the nonalert patient and not recommended for severe hypothermia)
    c) Active core: used to prevent core temperature afterdrop with active external rewarming
        (1) Warm (37 degrees C) IV infusion and heated (40 to 46 degrees C) oxygen as described previously
        (2) Warm gastric or peritoneal lavage, can be managed in emergency department
        (3) Inpatient measures for extreme hypothermia, including cardiopulmonary bypass, hemodialysis, and mediastinal irrigation

G. Administer medications
1. Naloxone: 0.8 to 2 mg IV push
2. Dextrose: 50 ml of 50% solution IV
3. Thiamine: 50 to 100 mg and multivitamins IV or IM for preexisting nutritional deficiencies
4. Tetanus immunization as indicated

Secondary intervention

A. Perform laboratory studies
1. Baseline: CBC, electrolytes, glucose, BUN, creatine, LDH, SGOT, SGPT, coagulation profile, serum calcium, serum magnesium
2. Others as indicated: alcohol and drug screens
3. ABGs; be sure temperature is correct

B. Obtain chest x-ray study

C. Serially monitor
1. Temperature via continuous rectal probe; keep alert for core temperature afterdrop
2. For fluid status
3. For electrolyte abnormalities
4. Frequently for neurological status

D. Treat associated problems and injuries as indicated

E. Examine for any evidence of frostbite

F. Rapidly rewarm any exposed extremity once core normothermia is stabilized

EVALUATION

I. Patient outcomes/criteria
   A. Return to normothermia
   B. Vital signs within normal limits
   C. Improved neurological status
   D. Normal sinus rhythm
   E. Electrolytes within normal limits

II. Document initial assessment data, emergency department interventio and the patient's response to treatment

III. If previous patient outcomes are not reached, the emergency nurse shoul reevaluate the interventions and change the plan of care accordingly

DISPOSITION

I. Admission criteria
   A. Any patient classified as moderately or severely hypothermic
   B. Severe frostbite

II. Discharge guidelines
   A. Evaluate living situation and make social service and visiting nurse r ferrals as appropriate
   B. Focus patient teaching on dangers of hypothermia as an environment hazard

CHAPTER 16

INFECTION: LOCALIZED

IPLICATIONS FOR ACTION

ocalized infection can range from a spontaneously occurring abscess to a life-reatening sepsis. Systemic illness should always be considered. Outpatient eatment mandates ability for self or family care.

SSESSMENT

i. Initial observation
  A. Location
  B. General appearance of site
I. Subjective assessment
  A. Mechanism of injury
  B. Onset and progression of signs of infection; duration
  C. Associated symptoms
    1. Chills and fever
    2. Tenderness or pain
    3. Loss of function, if applicable
  D. Medication allergies and tetanus immunization status
I. Objective assessment
  A. Vital signs, especially temperature
  B. Appearance of wound
    1. Erythema
    2. Streaking
    3. Drainage: amount, color, odor
    4. Edema
    5. Temperature of area
  C. Presence of sutures; approximation of wound edges

OSSIBLE NURSING DIAGNOSES/ANALYSIS

I. Comfort, alteration in: pain
II. Health maintenance, alteration in
II. Knowledge deficit (of wound care)

IV. Mobility, impaired physical
V. Noncompliance
VI. Nutrition, alteration in: less than body requirements
VII. Tissue perfusion, alteration in: peripheral

PLANNING

I. Priorities for care
   A. Systemic sepsis should be ruled out
   B. Local inflammatory process should be treated
   C. Discharge teaching
II. Differential management

Condition	Clinical Assessment	Management
CELLULITIS		
	Nonsuppurative inflammation of subcutaneous tissue; patient has erythema, edema, and pain; suppuration and necrosis may develop	Rest and antibiotics; admit for surgical drainage if rapid onset, extensive involvement, or potential of anaerobic organisms
LYMPHANGITIS		
	Inflammation of lymphatic pathways; may involve nodes; evidenced by red streaking	Rest involved part; admission to hospital for IV antibiotics (usually indicated)
ABSCESS		
	Inflamed tissue with localized suppuration	Incision and drainage; facial abscess often requires admission for IV antibiotics; danger of spread to intracranial area
BACTEREMIA		
	Bacteria transiently present in circulating blood; often no clinical indications	Usually not diagnosed
SEPTICEMIA		
	Bacteria and toxins in circulating blood cause diffuse infection; usually secondary to specific source; fever, chills; may progress to septic shock with hypotension, tachycardia, decreased level of consciousness	Perform blood cultures to identify organism; locate source of infection; perform hydration, give antibiotics; admission to hospital (refer to Chapter 27, Care Plan for Unresponsive Patient)

PLEMENTATION

Primary intervention

A. If sepsis is suspected:
   1. Initiate IV hydration with normal saline or lactated Ringer's
   2. Administer oxygen
   3. Obtain blood cultures and admission lab work
   4. Administer intravenous antibiotics, possibly steroids

B. Obtain laboratory data for localized inflammation
   1. Wound culture
   2. Gram stain if indicated

C. Incision and drainage of abscess are performed by physician

D. If symptoms progress from localized to systemic, refer to appropriate other care plan

Secondary intervention

A. Elevate, perform warm soaks as indicated

B. Give analgesics

C. Remove sutures and reopen wound as indicated

D. Apply dressing

ALUATION

. Patient outcomes/criteria
   A. Appearance of healing wound, e.g., absence of pus, redness, etc.
   B. Normal temperature
   C. Vital signs within normal limits

. Document initial assessment data, emergency department interventions, and patient's response to treatment

. If previous patient outcomes are not reached, the emergency nurse should reevaluate the interventions and change the plan of care accordingly

SPOSITION

Admission criteria

A. Patients with septicemia

B. Patients with a facial, hand, or foot abscess requiring IV antibiotic therapy

C. Patients requiring debridement in operating room

Discharge guidelines

A. Provide wound care instructions

B. Give medication instructions

C. Arrange follow-up checks or dressing changes

CHAPTER 17

MEDICAL CARDIO-PULMONARY ARREST

IMPLICATIONS FOR ACTION

Cardiopulmonary arrest—the most dramatic life-threatening event in eith the field or the emergency department—requires immediate, efficient, ar sophisticated medical and nursing intervention if there is to be any hope restoring life and brain function.

Specific standards of care and treatment modalities have been establishe for the treatment of cardiopulmonary arrest by the American Heart Associatic and the National Academy of Science National Research Council (1980) ar will serve as the foundation for this chapter.

The full scenario of treatment will be outlined, as if the arrest had o curred in the emergency department. However, with improved prehospit care systems—including citizens trained in cardiopulmonary resuscitatic (CPR) as well as paramedics—there will be increasing numbers of patien rescued from the field at the onset of their arrest. Once the patient arrives the emergency department, the primary concerns include: (1) if needed, co tinuing CPR and the restoration of cardiac and respiratory function or (2) th maintenance or prevention of deterioration from a life-sustaining rhyth achieved in the field.

ASSESSMENT

I. Initial observation
   A. Responsiveness: shake patient vigorously, call name
   B. Respiratory effort
   C. Presence of pulse: palpate carotid vessels
   D. Skin color and temperature

II. Subjective assessment (NOTE: Pertinent history should be obtained durir or after resuscitation efforts are under way, usually from family, field pe sonnel, or bystanders)

A. Activity at time of arrest
B. Pain preceding arrest
C. Downtime—time elapsed between collapse and initiation of care
D. Drugs or trauma involved (refer to appropriate standardized care plan)
E. Past medical history
   1. Previous myocardial infarction (MI) or cardiac disease
   2. Existing respiratory disease
   3. Medications and allergies
   4. Cardiac risk factors
      a) Smoking
      b) Hypertension
      c) Diabetes mellitus
      d) Positive family history
      e) Hypercholesteremia
      f) Obesity

I. Objective assessment
A. Airway
   1. Type
      a) None
      b) Esophageal obturator
      c) Endotracheal (ET) tube
   2. Adequacy
      a) Positioning
      b) Breath sounds: auscultate bilaterally
      c) ET tube placement: if any questions, visualize accurate placement with direct laryngoscopy
B. Breathing
   1. Any spontaneous respiratory effort by patient
   2. Assisted ventilation
      a) Mouth-to-mouth
      b) Bag-to-mouth
      c) Bag-to-ET tube
C. Circulation
   1. CPR in progress
      a) Adequate compressions: palpate carotid pulse
      b) Rate
   2. ECG monitoring: identify rhythm without CPR
D. Pupillary response

POSSIBLE NURSING DIAGNOSES/ANALYSIS

I. Breathing pattern, ineffective
II. Cardiac output, alteration in: decreased
III. Gas exchange, impaired
IV. Fear
V. Tissue perfusion, alteration in: cerebral, cardiopulmonary, renal, gast intestinal, peripheral
VI. Grieving, anticipatory (family or friends)

PLANNING

I. Priorities for care
   A. Adequate oxygenation
      1. Establishment or protection of established airway
      2. Administration of oxygen
   B. Effective CPR
   C. Establishment of patent intravenous access—preferably a central lin
   D. Restoration of effective cardiac functioning
      1. Treatment of life-threatening dysrhythmias
      2. Correction of acid/base balance
      3. Hemodynamic stabilization
      4. Prevention or treatment of recurrent dysrhythmias
II. Differential management

Condition	Clinical Assessment	Management
CARDIOVASCULAR ARREST		
Myocardial Infarction	May cause arrest or substernal or other chest pain, often described as a crushing sensation or pressure; may radiate to left arm, back/jaw, or neck; associated symptoms include nausea, vomiting, diaphoresis, and dyspnea; ECG may show ST segment elevation or depression, T wave inversion, dysrhythmias	Administer supplemental ox gen or ventilate if necessa provide intravenous acces perform cardiac monitorir administer prophylactic lidocaine (refer to boxes at end of care plan for do ages)

ondition	Clinical Assessment	Management
Cardiogenic shock	All the signs and symptoms of an acute MI plus pale, cool, clammy skin, dulled sensorium, tachycardia or bradycardia, an S_3 heart sound, weak or absent peripheral pulses, tachypnea, anxiety and restlessness, hypotension, and narrowing pulse pressure	In addition to the above measures, provide humidified oxygen by nonbreathing mask; adjust oxygen concentrations based on ABG analysis; if patient has chest pain, give morphine IV in small doses to control pain; if patient is hypovolemic, administer fluid challenge of lactated Ringer's until adequate outputs are achieved or signs of fluid overload appear; may administer vasoactive drug therapy; pneumatic antishock trousers may possibly be used; stabilize and arrange expedient transfer to ICU
rimary ysrhythmias		
Asystole	Patient is pulseless, comatose, with absent or gasping respirations	Perform CPR; intubate; administer central IV medications: epinephrine, sodium bicarbonate, calcium chloride, isoproterenol (refer to boxes at end of care plan for dosages); insert pacemaker (refer to appendix A for procedure and equipment)
Ventricular fibrillation	Patient is pulseless, comatose, with absent or gasping respirations	While defibrillator is charging, give patient precordial thump; then immediately defibrillate at 300-400 watt/sec; perform CPR; intubate; administer central IV medications: epinephrine, sodium bicarbonate, bretylium, or lidocaine (refer to boxes at end of care plan for dosages); repeat defibrillation; repeat medications; consider open-cardiac massage (refer to appendix A for procedure and equipment)

Condition	Clinical Assessment	Management
Ventricular tachycardia	Patient is often conscious with rapid pulse	Give precordial thump, estal lish IV access; administer medications: lidocaine, br tylium, procainamide, diaz pam (refer to boxes at en of care plan for dosages); vital signs deteriorate: cardiovert (if monitor shows upright R waves), defibrillate (if no R waves), insert pacemaker (refer to apper dix A for procedure and equipment)
	Patient is unconscious with or without a pulse	(As above); omit diazepam
Electro-mechanical dissociation	Patient is unconscious, no palpable pulse, but there is presence of electrical cardiac activity	Perform CPR; intubate; administer central IV medica tions: epinephrine, sodium bicarbonate, calcium chloride, isoproterenol (refer to boxes at end of care plan for dosages); check for tension pneumo thorax, cardiac tamponade volume depletion; conside open-cardiac massage
Severe bradycardia	Heart rate (HR) <50 or HR <60 along with hypotension or premature ventricular contractions (PVCs); patient may be unconscious or conscious, weak, disoriented	Administer medications: atropine, isoproterenol (refer to boxes at end of care plan for dosages), dopamine, norepinephrine; insert pacemaker
RESPIRATORY FAILURE*		
	(Refer to Chapter 22, Care Plan for Respiratory Distress for complete differential management)	
Ventilatory Insufficiency	Agonal, ineffective respirations or apnea	Oxygenate, intubate, treat un derlying respiratory proble
Airway Obstruction	Cyanosis, cardiac dysrhythmias resulting from hypoxia	Treat dysrhythmias that do n respond to increased oxygenation

ndition	Clinical Assessment	Management
ng Disease	(Refer to Chapter 22, Care Plan for Respiratory Distress)	
ng Trauma	(Refer to Chapter 34, Care Plan for Major Multiple Trauma)	
AUMA (cardiac trauma, hypovolemia, hypoxia)		
	(Refer to Chapter 34, Care Plan for Major Multiple Trauma for complete differential management)	
NTRAL NERVOUS SYSTEM DISRUPTION auma, drugs, infections, hypoxia)		
	(Refer to Chapter 27, Care Plan for Unresponsive Patient and other standardized care plans as indicated)	When associated with apnea, pulselessness, and cardiac dysrhythmias, resuscitation is the identical treatment given no matter the original etiology; however, additional treatment may be necessary (refer to appropriate standardized care plan according to suspected cause)

ost common cause of cardiopulmonary arrest in children.

PLEMENTATION

Primary intervention

A. Manage airway

1. Position patient: use head-tilt method to open airway; with suspected cervical spine injury, use jaw thrust method
2. Ventilate: initially, four quick breaths
   - *a*) Mouth-to-mouth with adults and children
   - *b*) Mouth-to-nose-and-mouth with infants or small children
   - *c*) Mask-to-mouth with ambu-bag
   - *d*) Mask-to-esophageal obturator with ambu-bag

B. Breathe until intubation is achieved
  1. Adult
    a) One breath every 5 seconds when doing two-person CPR
    b) Two breaths after every 15 compressions with one-person C
    c) 100% oxygen with ambu-bag
  2. Child
    a) One breath every 4 seconds
    b) 100% oxygen
  3. Infant (to 2 years of age)
    a) One breath every 3 seconds
    b) 100% oxygen

C. Intubate
  1. Gain complete control of airway: DO AS SOON AS POSSIBLE; if or nasal intubation cannot be quickly achieved, immediate cr thyrotomy must be performed (refer to appendix A for proced and equipment)
  2. Deliver high concentration of oxygen
  3. Most adults can be intubated with a size 7.5 to 8.5 endotracheal tu
  4. Children's sizes vary with age and size of child (rule of thumb: use tube closest to the size of the child's little finger, see table belo
  5. Check placement after intubation
    a) Auscultate lungs bilaterally
    b) Watch for rise and fall of chest
    c) Perform chest x-ray study after patient is stabilized
  6. Do not remove esophageal obturator airway (EOA) until after en tracheal tube has been placed

Approximate Age/Size Guide for Intubation of Children*

Age	Size
Newborn	2.5-3.5 mm
1 mo	3.5 mm
12 mo	4.0 mm
2-3 yr	4.5 mm
4-5 yr	6.0 mm
6-8 yr	6.5 mm
10-12 yr	7.0 mm
14 yr	7.5-8.5 mm

*Refer to box at end of care plan for pediatric continuous intravenous preparations and dosa

D. Establish circulation
   1. Perform external cardiac compressions: patient should be supine on a hard, flat surface
      a) Adult: use lower third of sternum and both hands; depress sternum 4 to 5 cm ($1\frac{1}{2}$-2 inches)
         (1) Rate of 60/min with two-person CPR
         (2) Rate of 80/min with one-person CPR
      b) Child: use lower half of sternum and heel of one hand; depress 2.5 to 3.8 cm (1 to $1\frac{1}{2}$ inches)
         (1) Rate of 80/min (same for one or two rescuers)
      c) Infant: use midsternum (ventricle lies higher than in adult) and index and middle finger; depress 1.3 to 2.5 cm ($\frac{1}{2}$-1 inch)
         (1) Rate of 100/min
   2. Establish venous access
      a) Peripheral: usually antecubital
      b) Central: subclavian or jugular; obtain portable chest x-ray study for proper placement and to rule out pneumothorax
      c) Interosseous for pediatrics
E. Recognize primary dysrhythmias*
   1. Asystole
   2. Ventricular fibrillation (Fig. 17-1)

*Refer to differential management section in this care plan for specific treatment.

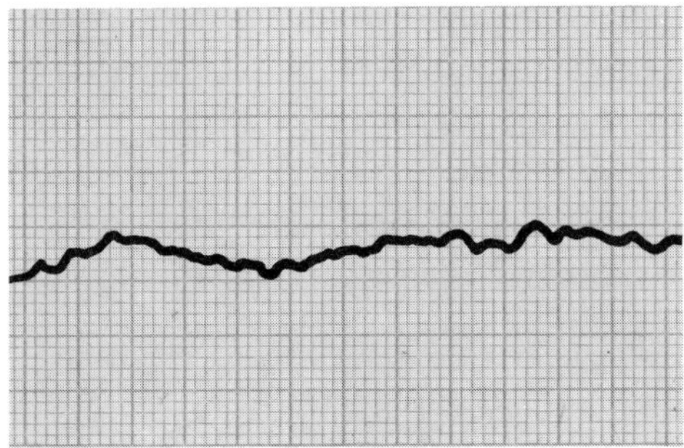

Fig. 17-1

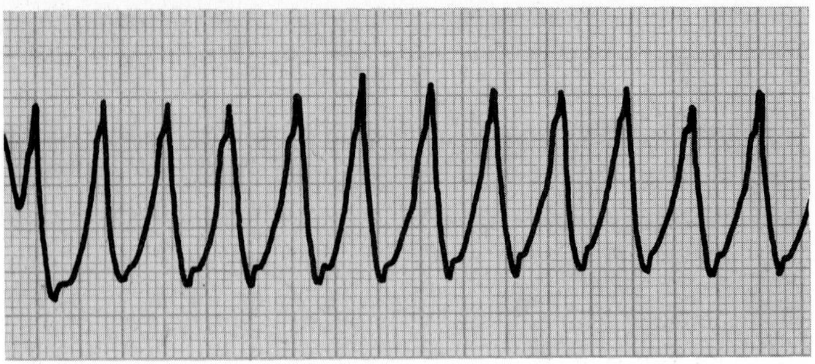

Fig. 17-2

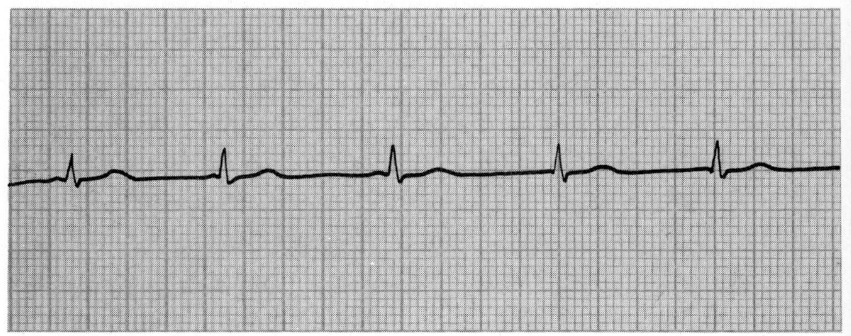

Fig. 17-3

3. Ventricular tachycardia (Fig. 17-2)
4. Electromechanical dissociation
5. Severe bradycardia (Fig. 17-3)

F. Recognize and treat secondary dysrhythmias; these dysrhythmias r arise after treatment of life-threatening primary dysrhythmias
1. Sinus tachycardia (Fig. 17-4)
   a) Try carotid sinus massage (CSM) if patient is symptomatic pulse is greater than 130
   b) Treat underlying cause of dysrhythmia

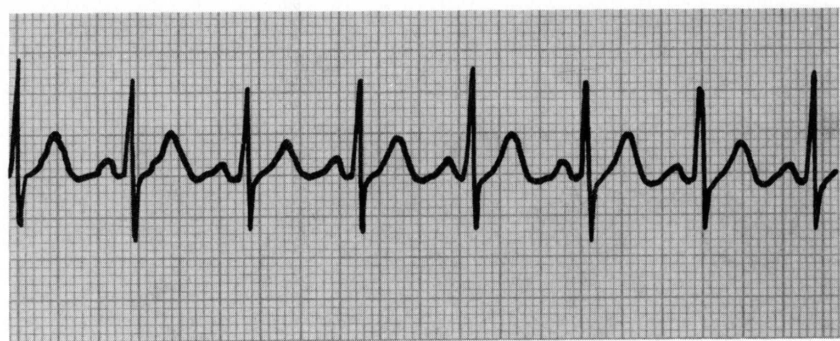

Fig. 17-4

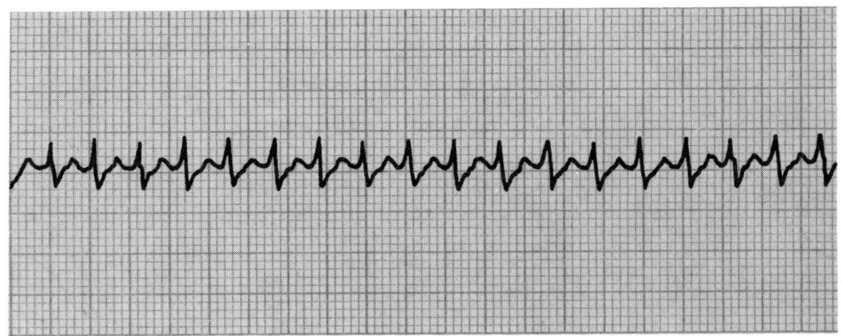

Fig. 17-5

2. Premature atrial contractions
   a) Usually caused by use of stimulants or sympathomimetic drugs
   b) Usually require no medications and will respond to oxygen
   c) May be sign of chronic lung disease
3. Paroxysmal atrial tachycardia (PAT) (Fig. 17-5)
   a) Use vagal maneuvers, carotid sinus massage, Valsalva maneuver, vomiting to convert
   b) Patient may need phenylephrine, edrophonium, propranolol, procainamide, lidocaine, verapamil, digoxin, sedatives (refer to boxes at end of care plan for dosages)
   c) May need to cardiovert with <100 joules if patient is symptomatic or does not respond to medications

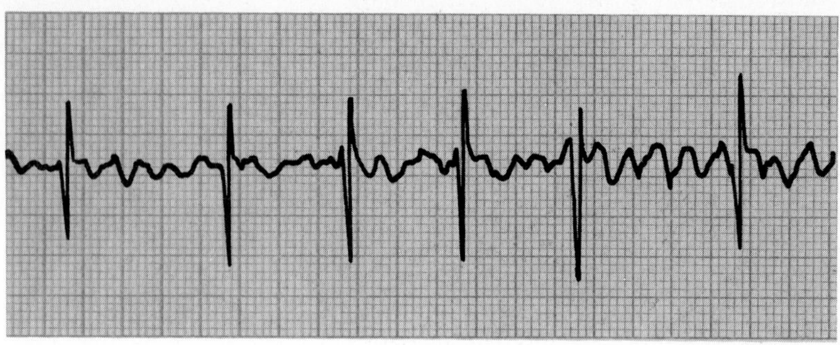

Fig. 17-6

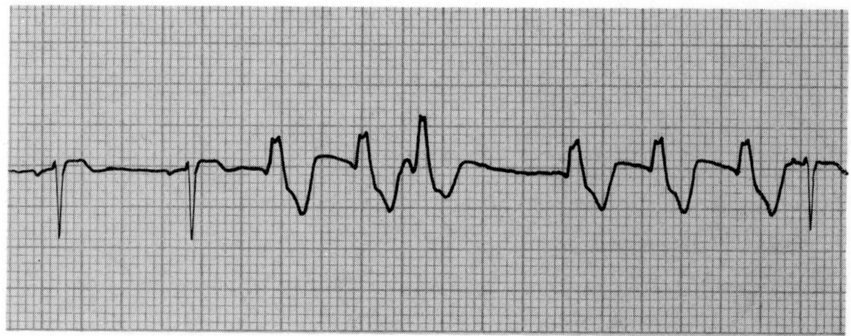

Fig. 17-7

4. Atrial fibrillation/flutter (Fig. 17-6)
   a) Administer digoxin, propranolol, procainamide, quinidine (ref
   to boxes at end of care plan for dosages)
   b) If patient is symptomatic, may need to perform cardioversio
   with <50 joules (use caution with chronic atrial fibrillation b
   cause of risk of embolization)
   c) With flutter, perform override pacing if cardioversion is unsu
   cessful
5. Premature ventricular contractions (PVCs) (Fig. 17-7)
   a) Administer lidocaine, procainamide, quinidine
   b) May need to use override pacing (refer to appendix A for proc
   dure and equipment)

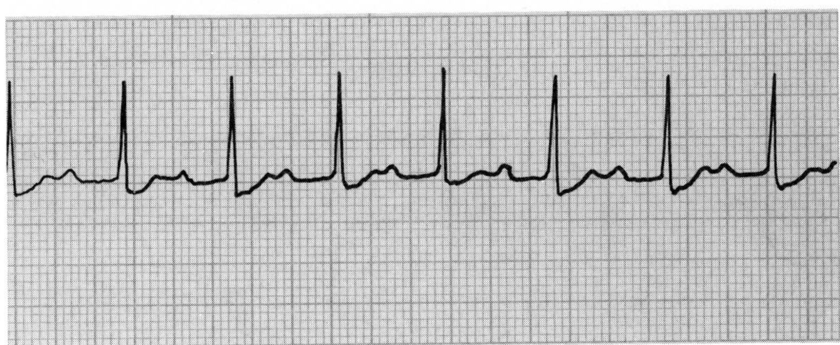

Fig. 17-8

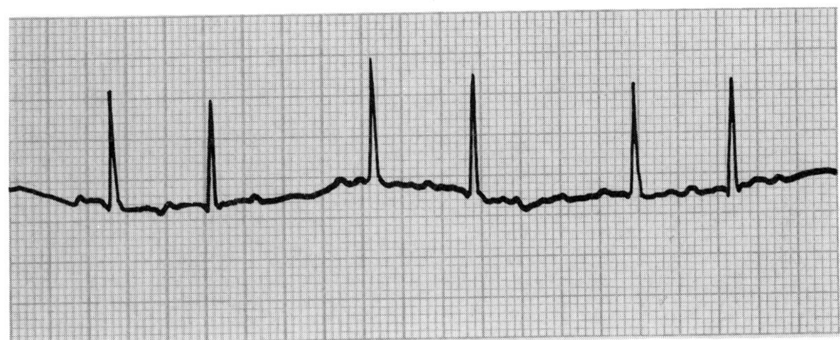

Fig. 17-9

6. Atrioventricular block (AV block)
   a) First-degree AV block (Fig. 17-8)
      (1) Observe for development of second- or third-degree AV block
      (2) May be caused by digitalis toxicity
   b) Second-degree AV block
      (1) Type I (Fig. 17-9)
         (*a*) Administer atropine if rate and blood pressure drop
         (*b*) Consider possible pacemaker insertion

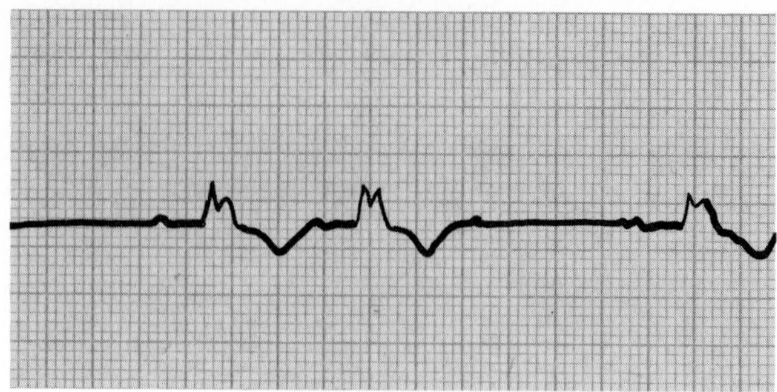

Fig. 17-10

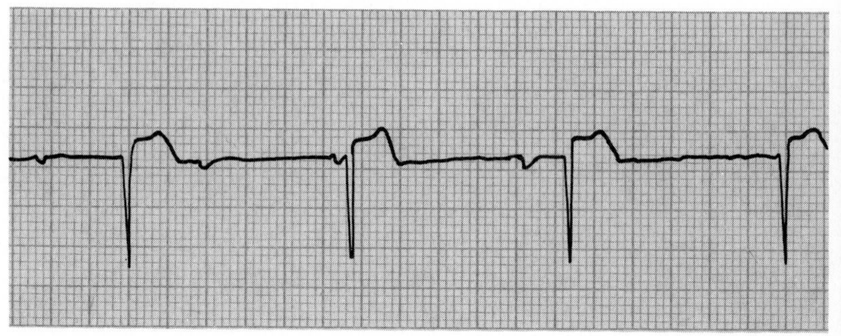

Fig. 17-11

(2) Type II (Fig. 17-10)
(*a*) Administer atropine if rate and blood pressure drop
(*b*) Consider pacemaker insertion
(*c*) Dangerous sign of heart disease and frequently dete orates to third-degree AV block

c) Third-degree AV block (Fig. 17-11)
(1) Administer atropine if rate and blood pressure drop
(2) Infuse with isoproterenol
(3) Insert pacemaker (treatment of choice)

G. Insert pacemaker (see appendix A for procedure and equipment)
1. Indications
a) Asystole
b) Severe bradydysrhythmias unresponsive to atropine or isopr terenol
c) Progressing second-degree or third-degree AV shock
d) Overdrive suppression of tachydysrhythmias

2. Preferred routes of insertion
   a) Internal jugular
   b) Subclavian
   c) Brachial
   d) Femoral
   e) Transthoracic

H. Perform pericardiocentesis (see appendix A for procedure and equipment)
   1. Indications: to relieve cardiac tamponade
   2. Assessment: increased CVP, pulsus paradoxus, respiratory distress, jugular vein distention, decreased blood pressure, ST-T wave abnormalities, electromechanical dissociation
   3. Treat with
      a) Volume infusion to increase ventricular filling pressures
      b) Pericardiocentesis: needle insertion into pericardial sac to draw off accumulated blood or fluid
      c) Treat resulting dysrhythmias or cause, i.e., hemorrhage or tension pneumothorax

I. Relieve tension pneumothorax (refer to Chapter 34, Care Plan for Major Multiple Trauma)

J. Perform open cardiac massage (refer to appendix A for procedure and equipment)
   1. Indications
      a) Cardiac arrest as a result of trauma
      b) Cardiac tamponade not relieved by pericardiocentesis
      c) Massive blood loss not responsive to fluid replacement
      d) Chest wall deformities that make external CPR ineffective
      e) Failure to respond to medical arrest protocols
   2. (Refer to Chapter 34, Care Plan for Major Multiple Trauma)

Secondary intervention

A. Once the patient has achieved a life-sustaining rhythm, primary concerns include
   1. Constant observation, including:
      a) Cardiac monitoring
      b) Frequent vital signs
      c) Maintenance of medication infusions
   2. Expedient transfer to intensive care unit (ICU)

B. For the conscious patient
   1. Explain briefly use of invasive equipment, including inability to talk because of ET tube
   2. Allow brief visit by family member

C. For the unconscious patient
   1. Take measures to protect the safety of the patient
   2. Allow brief visit by family member
D. Family needs
   1. Patient survival
      a) Provide explanations to family to alleviate anxiety/fear
      b) Allow brief visit by family after explaining presence of invasi equipment
   2. Patient death
      a) Provide privacy for grieving family
      b) Offer professional intervention, such as clergy, psychiatric me tal health services

EVALUATION

I. Patient outcomes/criteria
   A. Restored cardiac function
   B. Resolution of dysrhythmias
   C. Restored respiratory function
   D. Adequate central nervous system functioning
   E. Resuscitation efforts discontinued
II. Document initial assessment data, emergency department interventic and patient's response to treatment
III. If previous patient outcomes are not reached, the emergency nurse shou reevaluate the interventions and change the plan of care accordingly

DISPOSITION

I. Admission criteria (all patients who survive after a cardiac arrest will admitted to the intensive care unit)

DEFIBRILLATION/CARDIOVERSION GUIDELINES

Adult

Defibrillation: Begin with 200 to 300 watt/sec, increase energy with each attempt, not to exceed 400 watt/sec

Cardioversion: Use 200 watt/sec

Pediatric

Defibrillation: Use 2 watt/sec/kg

Use pediatric size paddles

CONTINUOUS INTRAVENOUS MEDICATIONS RECOMMENDED PREPARATIONS AND DOSAGE: PEDIATRIC

Dopamine
100 mg in 250 ml = 0.4 mg/ml
3-10-20 μg/kg/min
Start at 1 mgtt/kg/min

Isoproterenol
1 mg in 250 ml = 4 μg/ml
0.1-0.5 μg/kg
Start at 1 mgtt/kg/min and titrate

INTRAVENOUS MEDICATIONS: RECOMMENDED DOSES: PEDIATRIC

Atropine
1 mg = 1 ml
0.01 = 0.02 mg/kg
Maximum single dose: 0.5 mg

Bretylium tosylate
50 mg/ml
5-10 mg/kg

Calcium chloride
100 mg/ml = 10 ml = 1 gm (10% solution)
0.2 ml/kg of a 10% solution

Calcium glutamate
1 ml = 100 mg
100 mg/kg of a 10% solution

Epinephrine
1 mg/10 ml (1:10,000)
0.1 mg (1 ml/kg)

Glucose
1 ampule = 50 ml = 50 gm (1:1 solution)
2-4 mg/kg

Lidocaine
20 mg/ml = 5 ml = 100 mg
1 mg/kg

Sodium bicarbonate
1 ampule = 44.6 mEq = 50 cc
1 mEq/kg every 10 min

CONTINUOUS INTRAVENOUS MEDICATIONS RECOMMENDED PREPARATIONS AND DOSAGE: ADULT

Aramine
1 ml = 10 mg; mix 10-25 mg/500 ml = 0.2-0.5 mg/1 ml
Titrate to blood pressure
Start at 60-120 mgtt/min

Bretylium
4 ampules (2 gm) in 500 ml = 4 mg/ml
4 mg/min = 60 mgtt/min
3 mg/min = 45 mgtt/min
2 mg/min = 30 mgtt/min
1 mg/min = 15 mgtt/min

Dobutrex
10 ml = 250 mg; mix 500 mg in 500 ml = mg/ml
Dose = 2.5-10.0 μg/kg/min
1 mg/min = 60 mgtt/min
0.75 mg/min = 45 mgtt/min
0.50 mg/min = 30 mgtt/min
0.25 mg/min = 15 mgtt/min

Dopamine
5 ml = 400 mg; mix 400 mg in 250 ml = 1600 mg/ml
Dose = 2-10 μg/kg/min; titrate to blood pressure
1400 μg/min = 52 mgtt/min
700 μg/min = 26 mgtt/min
350 μg/min = 13 mgtt/min
140 μg/min = 5 mgtt/min

Isuprel
5 ml = 1 mg; mix 2 mg in 500 ml = 4 μg/ml
Dose = 2-20 μg/min; titrate to heart rate
Start at 60 mgtt/min (1 ml)

Levophed
4 ml = 8 mg; mix in 500 ml = 16 μg/ml
Titrate to blood pressure
Start at 120-180 mgtt/min (2 to 3 ml)

Lidocaine
Mix 2 gm in 500 ml = 4 mg/ml
4 mg/min = 60 mgtt/min
3 mg/min = 45 mgtt/min
2 mg/min = 30 mgtt/min
1 mg/min = 15 mgtt/min

INTRAVENOUS MEDICATIONS: RECOMMENDED DOSES (ACLS): ADULT

Atropine
0.1 mg/ml = 1 mg/10 ml
Total dose: 2 mg

Bretylium tosylate
50 mg/ml
5-10 mg/kg rapidly every 15-30 min
Total dose: 30 mg/kg
(Follow with continuous intravenous infusion)

Calcium chloride
100 mg/ml = 10 ml = 1 gm
0.5-1 gm of a 10% solution every 10 min

Epinephrine
1 mg/10 ml (1:10,000)
0.5-1 mg every 10 min

Propranolol
1 mg/ml
1 mg slowly, every 5 min
Total dose: 3-5 mg

Lidocaine
20 mg/ml = 5 ml = 100 mg
1 mg/kg as first dose
Repeat bolus every 5-10 min with 0.5 mg/kg
Total dose: 300 mg
(Follow with continuous intravenous infusion)

Procainamide
1 ml = 100 mg
0.2-1 gm slowly

Sodium bicarbonate
1 ampule = 44.6 mEq = 50 cc
1 mEq/kg as first dose
Repeat one half of first dose every 10 min or according to ABGs

CHAPTER 18

NAUSEA AND VOMITING

IMPLICATIONS FOR ACTION

Symptoms of nausea and vomiting are common with many conditions of a tered health. This care plan outlines immediate care of the patient and pr vides referral to other appropriate care plans.

ASSESSMENT

I. Initial observation
  A. Skin color
  B. Patient's stance
II. Subjective assessment
  A. Frequency, amount, and color of emesis, with or without nausea; reli with vomiting
  B. Associated symptoms
    1. Fever, chills
    2. Diarrhea, obstipation
    3. Abdominal pain: exact location, character, and duration
    4. Flank pain, dysuria
    5. Vaginal discharge or bleeding
III. Objective assessment
  A. Orthostatic vital signs
  B. Rectal temperature, if unable to obtain an accurate oral temperature
  C. Skin turgor, moistness of mucous membranes
  D. Bowel sounds present or absent, frequency
  E. Abdominal distention
  F. Description of emesis, if observed

POSSIBLE NURSING DIAGNOSES/ANALYSIS

I. Comfort, alteration in: pain
II. Fluid volume deficit, actual or potential
III. Nutrition, alteration in: less than body requirements

ANNING

Priorities for care

A. Fluid and electrolyte management

B. Allowing gastrointestinal system to rest

C. Diagnosis of underlying cause

Differential management

nditions	Clinical Assessment (Causes)	Management
STROINTESTINAL SYSTEM		
	Gastritis, gastroenteritis, liver or gallbladder disease, pancreatitis, bowel obstruction, food poisoning, appendicitis	Manage fluid and electrolytes (refer to Chapter 1, Care Plan for Abdominal Pain and Chapter 11, Care Plan for Gastrointestinal Bleeding)
EUROLOGICAL SYSTEM		
	Meningitis, intracranial bleeding, migraine headaches, tumor, increased intracranial pressure	(Refer to Chapter 12, Care Plan for Headache)
ETABOLIC SYSTEM		
	Diabetes, adrenal failure, myxedema, hypercalcemia, hypokalemia	Obtain laboratory data to isolate etiology of metabolic disturbance
YPEREMESIS GRAVIDARUM		
	Occurs in first trimester of pregnancy; ketones may be present in urine	Initiate IV hydration until patient is able to tolerate oral fluids; limited medications only should be given to pregnant women
ISCELLANEOUS CAUSES		
	Cardiac etiology: digitalis toxicity, myocardial infarction	Monitor digoxin level; (refer to Chapter 4, Care Plan for Chest Pain)
	Other: intussusception; pyloric stenosis; Meckel's diverticulum	(Refer to Chapter 1, Care Plan for Abdominal Pain and Chapter 7, Care Plan for Dysuria)
	Anorexia nervosa	Arrange psychiatric therapy and fluid and electrolyte management

IMPLEMENTATION

I. Primary intervention
  A. Administer IV: normal saline or lactated Ringer's for orthostasis, co
     tinuous vomiting, hematemesis, or for patient with acutely ill appea
     ance; use slower IV rate for patients with increased intracranial pressu
  B. Check emesis for blood
  C. Patient should be NPO; insert nasogastric tube for hematemesis, acu
     abdominal condition, pancreatitis, or obstruction
  D. Obtain laboratory data
    1. Hematocrit
    2. Electrolytes; complete blood count (CBC), especially if patient
       febrile; amylase if abdominal pain is present
    3. Urine for ketones, specific gravity
    4. Other tests to rule out metabolic causes (e.g., glucose, drug levels

II. Secondary intervention
  A. Administer medications
    1. Potassium replacement as indicated; usually given IV since oral rou
       often is not tolerated
    2. Antiemetics or anticholinergic drugs for prolonged vomiting
  B. Accurately monitor intake and output
  C. Institute comfort measures
    1. Moisten patient's lips; ice chips increase ileus in some patients
    2. Use glycerin swabs
  D. Repeat orthostatic vital signs after each 500 ml to 1000 ml of IV flui
     observe for fluid overload in elderly: presence of rales, tachycardi
     shortness of breath

EVALUATION

I. Patient outcomes/criteria
  A. Resolution of orthostasis
  B. Ability to tolerate oral fluids
  C. Continued presence of associated symptoms

II. Document initial assessment data, emergency department intervention
    and patient's response to treatment

III. If previous patient outcomes are not reached, the emergency nurse shou
     reevaluate the interventions and change the plan of care accordingly

ISPOSITION

Admission criteria

A. Patient may require admission if unable to retain oral fluids

B. Etiology of nausea or vomiting may warrant admission

Discharge guidelines

A. Give instructions for treating the cause of nausea and vomiting

B. Advise patient to return if symptoms persist or worsen

CHAPTER 19

PEDIATRIC EMERGENCIES (RESPIRATORY DISTRESS, FEVER, SEIZURE)

IMPLICATIONS FOR ACTION

The pediatric care plan includes a selection of common pediatric conditio treated in an emergency department. Additional information pertaining pediatrics is interspersed among the other care plans, such as those on Medic Arrest, Seizure, Poisoning, and Trauma. The following protocol outlines t priorities for care of a pediatric emergency.

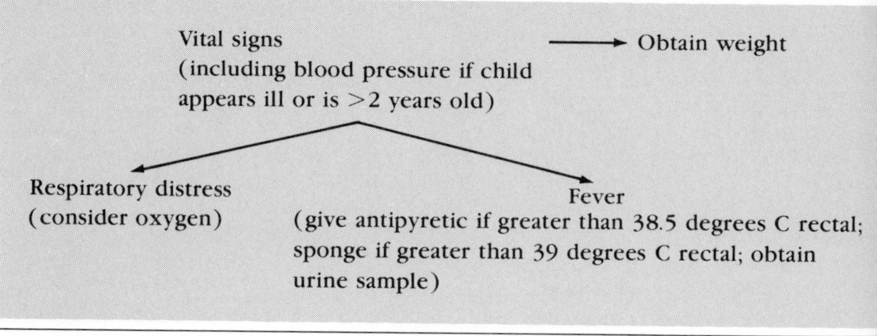

ASSESSMENT

I. Initial observation
   A. Skin color
   B. Respiratory effort
   C. Sound of cry

D. Level of activity or alertness

E. General appearance

I. Subject assessment

A. Description of complaint

1. Time of onset
2. Change in behavior or activity (listen carefully to parent)
3. Complaints or indications of pain such as tugging at ear
4. Appetite and recent nutritional intake

B. Associated information

1. Home interventions: time and dosage of medications
2. Response to treatment measures
3. Sick siblings or playmates

C. Past medical history

1. Previous illness
2. Known allergies
3. Medications
4. Immunization status and past reactions; recent injections

I. Objective assessment

A. Vital signs

1. Refer to table below for normal values
2. Temperature, pulse, and respirations should be obtained in all children; blood pressure should be obtained in children over 2 years and infants who are acutely ill
3. Respiratory rate and effort, nasal flaring, intercostal or sternal retraction, or use of accessory muscles should be assessed
4. Skin color and temperature
5. Weight is used to calculate medication dosage and should be obtained in all children; may be a clue to magnitude of dehydration

ediatric Vital Signs

Age	Pulse	Respirations	Blood Pressure	
			Systolic	Diastolic
nfants	110-160	30-60	60-100	40-70
2 years	100-140	28-36	70-110	40-70
4 years	80-110	24-28	80-110	40-80
6 years	80-110	22-28	80-110	50-80
8-10 years	70-100	20-28	70-120	50-80
0-12 years	60- 90	14-18	90-140	50-70

B. Clinical signs of dehydration
   1. Decreased urine output (ask for diaper count or trips to bathroom)
   2. Lack of tears when crying
   3. Dry mucous membranes
   4. Reduced skin turgor
   5. Sunken fontanelles in infants
   6. In older children, orthostatic vital signs may be significant

C. Mental status and level of activity
   1. Alertness
   2. If older child, response to questions
   3. If infant, response to environment and stimulus
   4. Listlessness, lethargy, or irritability

POSSIBLE NURSING DIAGNOSES/ANALYSIS

I. Airway clearance, ineffective
II. Bowel elimination, alteration in: diarrhea
III. Breathing pattern, ineffective
IV. Communication, impaired: verbal
V. Comfort, alteration in: pain
VI. Fear
VII. Fluid volume deficit, actual
VIII. Gas exchange, impaired
IX. Injury: potential for
X. Knowledge deficit (of common childhood illnesses and at-home care)
XI. Nutrition, alteration in: less than body requirements
XII. Parenting, alteration in: actual or potential
XIII. Tissue perfusion, alteration in: cerebral, cardiopulmonary, gastrointestinal

PLANNING

I. Priorities for care
   A. Airway management
   B. Hydration
   C. Identifying cause of infection
   D. Parental education

II. Differential management (this section is designed to outline only the most common *nontraumatic* pediatric problems seen in the emergency department)

Pediatric Emergencies (Respiratory Distress, Fever, Seizure)

ndition	Clinical Assessment	Management
SPIRATORY DISTRESS		
thma	Precipitating events include allergic reaction, infection, emotional stress; symptoms include labored respirations, inspiratory and expiratory wheezing, chest retractions, nasal flaring, tachypnea, and tachycardia; the child with severe distress may not be moving enough air to produce audible wheezing	Administer humidified oxygen 4-6 L/min by mask or cannula 1. Bronchodilator therapy: Epinephrine 1:1000 0.01 ml/kg S.Q. up to 0.3 ml (do not give if heart rate >180/min) 2. Nebulizer treatment: a. Isoetharine (Bronkosol) 0.25-0.5 ml/3 ml in normal saline b. Metaproterenol (Alupent) 0.3 ml/2.5 ml in normal saline c. Sus-Phrine (1:200) may be given for long-acting bronchodilator effect at 0.005 ml/kg S.Q. If patient does not respond to above bronchodilator therapy, aminophylline is initiated; obtain serum level if child is presently taking it; loading dose = 6 mg/kg IV over 20 minutes; maintenance infusion 0.8-1.2 mg/kg per hour
eumonia	Nonspecific symptoms in infants: decreased activity, vomiting, anorexia, fever, tachypnea	Administer humidified oxygen if respiratory distress is present; severe distress will necessitate intubation and arterial blood gas
	Older children: fever, tachypnea, cough, abdominal discomfort with vomiting, pleuritic chest pain, malaise	Perform complete blood count, blood cultures, chest x-ray study, hydration, suctioning; administer antibiotics if bacterial or mycoplasmic etiology is suspected

Condition	Clinical Assessment	Management
Croup (Laryngotracheobronchitis)	Inflammatory response of respiratory tract, usually caused by a virus; common age 6 months to 3 years; symptoms typically begin at night and include barklike cough, hoarseness, inspiratory and expiratory stridor, low grade fever, possibly labored respirations with retraction; child may improve on way to hospital	Differentiate from epiglottitis; (refer to management of epiglottitis below) 1. Mild croup: use humidified air, either cold mist or steam; if child is at home, take outside or turn on shower in bathroom 2. Stridor at rest or increased respiratory distress requires hospital care; continued humidification; administer racemic epinephrine 0.5 ml (2% solution) in 2.5 ml normal saline for nebulizer treatment; these children require admission because of rebound effects; severe respiratory distress requires intubation and oxygenation; other management includes hydration and possibly steroids
Epiglottitis	Usually bacterial infection, may occur at any age but peaks at 2-5 years; rapid onset of symptoms throughout the day, including muffled voice, drooling (because of dysphagia), high fever, inspiratory stridor; usually no cough; child often leans forward to maximize air movement; restlessness, anxiety; edema may progress, resulting in complete airway obstruction	DO NOT LEAVE CHILD UNATTENDED To differentiate from croup: 1. If severe respiratory distress or obstruction does not exist, obtain portable lateral, soft tissue neck x ray to visualize epiglottitis 2. Physician will visualize epiglottitis in controlled environment with intubation equipment and experienced personnel present

ndition	Clinical Assessment	Management
iglottitis—nt'd		Once diagnosis is made or if severe respiratory distress or obstruction is present, intubation, or, if necessary, surgical airway management is indicated; provide humidified oxygen; establish intravenous access for hydration and antibiotics; laboratory data should include complete blood count and blood cultures (NOTE: Laboratory tests and IV access are to be obtained only after airway control is obtained; the initial hypoxia should be reversed with oxygen, while intubation equipment is readied; do not make child worse by causing crying from IV or blood drawing until after the airway is controlled)
reign Body	Tracheobronchial foreign body (FB) causes stridor, respiratory distress, cough; may cause complete obstruction	Obstruction requires immediate airway management by manual thrusts and backblows as outlined by American Heart Association
	Esophageal foreign body with compression to respiratory tract causes cough, dysphasia, respiratory distress	Visualize with laryngoscopy and remove foreign body with Magill forceps, clamp, or bronchoscopy; cricothyrotomy may be required to bypass obstruction (refer to appendix A for procedure and equipment); initiate oxygen therapy as soon as possible; the child with no or mild distress should have chest x-ray or soft tissue lateral neck studies to locate foreign body; endoscopy may be required for esophageal foreign body

Condition	Clinical Assessment	Management
FEVER		
	Fever in child is defined as rectal temperature >38 degrees C; fever in child <3 months old requires workup and probably hospitalization to rule out sepsis; common causes of fever in children: otitis media, pneumonia, strep throat, meningitis, urinary tract infection, reaction to immunizations; assess hydration status, recent eating habits, urinary output, orthostatic vital signs in older children; there may be CNS symptoms of irritability, headache, confusion, nuchal rigidity; febrile seizures most commonly occur between 6 months and 3 years	Undress child and institute antipyretic therapy: acetaminophen 10-15 mg/kg for rectal temperature >38 degrees C; obtain urine sam ple (apply urine bag in infant); perform hydration: or or intravenous; physical examination by physician; laboratory test may be needed to isolate cause: EN exam, urinalysis, white bloo cell count; possibly chest x ray, blood cultures, lumba puncture; DO NOT GIVE ASPIRIN IF VIRAL SYNDROME IS SUSPECTED
SEIZURE		
	Consider the following causes in Neonates: Injury at birth (anoxia), infection (meningitis), metabolic disorders Children: Febrile seizures (6 months to 3 years), head trauma, infection, idiopathic epilepsy, metabolic disorders, poisoning, tumors	(Refer to Chapter 23, Care Pla for Seizures for managemen guidelines)
TRAUMA		
	(Refer to Care Plans for Chapter 34, Major Multiple Trauma; Chapter 36, Orthopedic Injuries; and Chapter 29, Child Abuse)	

ndition	Clinical Assessment	Management
STROINTESTINAL DISORDERS		
stroenteritis	Presence of vomiting and diarrhea; anorexia; abdominal pain; listlessness; assess frequency, character, presence of blood; assess change in food or formula, recent travelling; possibility of toxic ingestion	Initiate hydration: intravenous if child cannot tolerate oral intake; obtain laboratory data: complete blood count if child is febrile or there is presence of abdominal pain, urinalysis if there is abdominal pain, electrolytes and glucose if prolonged vomiting or diarrhea, stool culture
pendicitis	Classical presentation is periumbilical pain subsequently localizing to RLQ, but patient may have only vague abdominal pain; accompanied with fever, malaise, nausea, vomiting, anorexia; may progress to peritonitis and sepsis if not treated	Obtain laboratory data: complete blood count; perform intravenous access and administer antibiotics; prepare child and family for surgery

IPLEMENTATION

Primary intervention

A. Follow guidelines in differential management section

B. Manage airway for respiratory distress, obstruction, suspected croup or epiglottitis, cyanosis
   1. Apply oxygen 4 to 6 L/min via mask or cannula
   2. Ventilate if child is in respiratory arrest
   3. Prepare intubation equipment and suction (refer to Chapter 17, p. 104, for pediatric intubation information)

C. Perform hydration
   1. Apply urine collection bag on any infant who has fever, abdominal pain
   2. Offer oral fluids if child is able to tolerate them, such as clear liquids, electrolyte solutions, formula

3. If parenteral fluids are required for hydration
    a) Use dextrose 5% and normal saline, or dextrose 5% and lactate Ringer's, or dextrose 5% and 0.45 normal saline
    b) Administer 20 ml/kg over 45 to 60 minutes to treat mild de hydration (20 to 30 ml/kg rapidly if child is in hypovolemi shock or has extreme dehydration)
    c) Use a Buritrol or Soluset on intravenous tubing to avoid potenti volume overload
    d) Carefully monitor intake and output
    e) Isolate source of infection; laboratory tests are outlined in diffe ential management section

II. Secondary intervention
  A. Obtain serial vital signs and assessments
  B. Offer reassurance and support to patient and family
  C. Assess learning needs of parents and provide careful teaching

EVALUATION

I. Patient outcomes/criteria
  A. Improved color and breath sounds
  B. Normal vital signs for age group
  C. Toleration of oral fluids
  D. Parents able to describe or demonstrate understanding of discharg information

II. Document initial assessment, emergency department intervention, and pa tient and family's response to treatment

III. If previous patient outcomes are not reached, the emergency nurse shoul reevaluate the interventions and change the plan of care accordingly

DISPOSITION

I. Admission criteria
  A. Child who is unable to tolerate oral fluids
  B. Child who has received racemic epinephrine treatment for croup
  C. Child less than 8 weeks old with fever for sepsis workup
  D. Continued respiratory distress
  E. Need for intravenous antibiotics

II. Discharge guidelines
  A. Provide careful teaching to parents (refer to discharge instructions i appendix E)
  B. Discuss follow-up arrangements

CHAPTER 20

POISONING

IPLICATIONS FOR ACTION

ie patient with acute poisoning offers a challenge to the emergency depart-ent team. Multidrug ingestions are common, resulting in a mixture of symp-ms. An alert, seemingly stable patient may rapidly deteriorate because of stemic absorption of a significant poison. If the ingestion is intentional, be-vioral problems such as denial or active resentment of treatment may sur-ce.

Priorities are airway and circulatory management along with administra-on of antidotes and antagonists if available. Steps to enhance removal of the xin are then performed (refer to Care Plans for Chapter 31, Eye Injuries; iapter 33, Inhalation Injuries; Chapter 40, Radioactive Contamination; and iapter 41, Wound Management for further information on poisonings).

SSESSMENT

. Initial observation
  - A. Respiratory status
  - B. Level of consciousness
  - C. Behavior
    1. Withdrawn
    2. Agitated
    3. Combative

. Subjective assessment
  - A. Description of incident
    1. Name and amount of substance(s) ingested
    2. Duration of time since ingestion
    3. Vomiting after ingestion
    4. Home remedies
  - B. Reason for ingestion
    1. Accidental
    2. Suicidal
    3. Recreational

C. Family, witnesses, and paramedics should be interviewed since patient's account of incident may not be honest

D. Associated symptoms
   1. Abdominal pain
   2. Nausea, vomiting, diarrhea, hematemesis
   3. Dysphagia
   4. Drowsiness or restlessness
   5. Drooling, salivation
   6. Palpitations
   7. Dry mouth
   8. Dyspnea, cough
   9. Hallucinations
   10. Visual disturbances/photophobia
   11. Seizure

E. Past history
   1. Pertinent medical and mental health history
   2. Current medications and recreational drug use
   3. Alcohol intake

F. Assessment of patient's acceptance of treatment

G. Evaluation of need for physical restraints in view of patient's behavior or concern for patient leaving before treatment

III. Objective assessment

A. Vital signs
   1. Blood pressure, pulse, temperature
   2. Respiratory rate and quality

B. Neurological status
   1. Level of consciousness
   2. Orientation
   3. Pupil size and reactivity
   4. Presence of seizure activity
   5. Motor weakness/ataxia
   6. Gag reflex
      a) Never a reliable indicator of neurological status
      b) Normally absent in many individuals
      c) Rely instead on clinical assessment of patient

C. Skin color, temperature, diaphoresis

D. Drug containers (note date prescription filled and amount missing) help to identify substance and amount ingested

POSSIBLE NURSING DIAGNOSES/ANALYSIS

I. Airway clearance, ineffective
II. Anxiety
III. Breathing pattern, ineffective
IV. Cardiac output, alteration in: decreased
V. Coping, ineffective individual
VI. Fluid volume deficit: actual or potential
VII. Gas exchange, impaired
VIII. Grieving
IX. Injury: poisoning, potential for
X. Knowledge deficit (potential for poisoning)
XI. Noncompliance
XII. Oral mucous membranes, alteration in
XIII. Self-concept, disturbance in: body image, self-esteem, role performance, personal identity
XIV. Sensory-perceptual alteration: visual, auditory
XV. Social isolation
XVI. Thought processes, alteration in
XVII. Tissue perfusion, alteration in: cerebral, cardiopulmonary, renal, gastrointestinal, peripheral
XVIII. Violence, potential for: self-directed or directed at others

PLANNING

I. Priorities for care
   A. Airway management
   B. Circulatory management
   C. Removing and preventing absorption of toxin
   D. Prevention of additional self-harm
II. Differential management (NOTE: The management interventions in the table are specific to the toxin; all patients require assessment and appropriate treatment for respiratory and hemodynamic compromise; TREAT THE PATIENT—NOT THE POISON)

Type	Clinical Assessment	Management
ACETAMINOPHEN		
	Patient may have no symptoms or nausea, vomiting, anorexia; hepatotoxicity 24-36 hours after ingestion evidenced by increased SGOT, right abdominal pain, hypoglycemia, or abnormal clotting studies	Emesis or lavage; usually hol charcoal administration un acetaminophen level obtained; some evidence that charcoal may interfere wit acetylcysteine treatment; obtain acetaminophen leve 4 hours or more after inge tion; if drug levels are not rapidly available, treat empirically if size of ingestion is potentially toxic; if in toxic range, administer acetylcysteine (NAC or Mycomyst) orally or through nasogastric tube; load: 140 mg/kg, then 70 mg/kg q4 hours for 17 doses
ACIDS AND ALKALIS		
	Patient may have caustic oral, esophageal, and gastric burns; bloody emesis; abdominal or chest pain; hypotension and hemolysis; inhalation may result in dyspnea and pulmonary edema; eventually esophageal strictures, gastric outlet obstruction or perforation, pneumonia may develop	DO NOT INDUCE EMESIS; gastric aspiration recommended immediately following acid ingestion, contraindicated in alkali ingestion; give milk or wat orally; charcoal administra tion not of value; obtain electrolytes
ALCOHOLS		
Ethanol	Progression of symptoms: diminished fine motor control, altered sensation, impaired coordination and judgment, delayed reaction time, ataxia, uninhibited behavior, lethargy, coma, respiratory depression; commonly taken with other drug ingestions	Manage airway; lavage if patient has consumed larg amount of ethanol just before arrival in the department (refer to Chapter 2, Care Plan for Alcohol Into ication)

pe	Clinical Assessment	Management
hylene Glycol	Signs and symptoms of intoxication: epigastric pain, vomiting; patient may develop acidosis, pulmonary edema, seizures, coma, and renal failure	Provide intravenous ethanol infusion; dialysis
opropyl cohol	Signs and symptoms of intoxication: epigastric pain, vomiting	Manage airway
ethanol	Signs and symptoms of intoxication: severe photophobia, tachypnea, epigastric pain, vomiting, seizures, acidosis; may cause blindness	Provide intravenous ethanol infusion; dialysis
IPHETAMINES		
	Agitation, irritability, insomnia, tachycardia, hypertension, hallucinations, paranoia, aggression, seizures, coma	Emesis or lavage followed by charcoal and cathartic; may require sedation with haloperidol
ITICHOLINERGICS		
	Agitation, dilated pupils, warm dry skin, tachycardia, hypertension, hallucinations, urinary retention, seizures, coma	Emesis or lavage followed by charcoal and cathartic 1. Physostigmine: a. Adult: 2 mg IV (1 mg/min); may repeat every 20 minutes for total of 6 mg b. Pediatric: 0.5 mg IV (0.5 mg/min); may repeat every 5 minutes for total of 2 mg
RBITURATES		
	Patient stuporous to comatose; respiratory depression to arrest, hypotension	Lavage followed by charcoal and cathartic; alkaline diuresis for phenobarbital ingestion: sodium bicarbonate 1-2 mEq/kg in 1000 ml dextrose 5% or dextrose 5% .25 normal saline to keep urine pH 7.5; maintain urine output at 3-6 ml/kg/hour

Type	Clinical Assessment	Management
BENZODIAZEPINE		
	Ataxia, lethargy, slurred speech; patient may develop hypotension, respiratory depression; increased CNS depression when combined with other drugs such as alcohol or barbiturates	Lavage followed by charcoal and cathartic
COCAINE		
	Restlessness, agitation, tachycardia and other arrhythmias, diaphoresis, hypertension, dilated pupils; may progress to hypotension, coma, seizures, respiratory or cardiac arrest	Most exposures via nasal inhalation or intravenousl if oral dose, emesis or lava followed by charcoal and cathartic; surgical removal may be warranted if cocaine-filled bags are swallowed; propranolol us ally drug of choice for dys rhythmias
CYANIDE		
	Rapid progression of symptoms: confusion, headache; initially hypertension with bradycardia followed by hypotension, tachycardia, tachypnea, cyanosis, pulmonary edema, coma, and death	Lilly Cyanide Antidote Kit: 1. Have patient breathe amyl nitrite pearle for of every 60 seconds un sodium nitrite is administered 2. Sodium nitrite IV: a. Adult: 300 mg over 3-5 minutes (10 ml 3% solution) b. Pediatric: 0.2-0.3 mg/kg, up to 10 ml 3. Sodium thiosulfate IV: a. Adult: 12.5 gm (50 of 25% solution) b. Pediatric: 1.65 ml/k up to 12.5 gm 4. Repeat 1/2 dose of step (2) and (3) in 30 min symptoms recur

pe	Clinical Assessment	Management
DROCARBONS		
	Nausea, vomiting, abdominal pain; dyspnea and coughing indicative of aspiration; lethargy, coma, seizures, cardiac arrhythmias and cyanosis; high incidence of pulmonary edema and hemorrhagic pneumonitis because of aspiration	Gastric emptying either by emesis or lavage is controversial because of increased risk of aspiration; decision will be based on amount ingested, viscosity of substance, and patient's clinical status; value of charcoal and cathartic administration also controversial; obtain chest x-ray study—signs of chemical pneumonitis may not appear for 6-8 hours
ON		
	Phase I: Nausea, vomiting, hematemesis, diarrhea, abdominal pain, lethargy, hypotension Phase II: Cessation of symptoms Phase III: Hypotension, acidosis, fever, hypoxia; may progress to hemorrhage, renal failure, and death Phase IV: Possible hepatic necrosis	Emesis or lavage followed by cathartic; obtain serum iron and total iron-binding capacity; perform deferoxamine chelation for 10-15 mg/kg/hour; initiate IV infusion in dextrose 5% for 8 hours; watch for orange-colored urine indicating chelation; obtain chest and abdominal x-ray studies to identify location and amount of iron; may require surgical removal of iron bezoar
SERGIC ACID (LSD)		
	Anxiety, restlessness, tachycardia, hypertension, hyperthermia, dilated pupils; auditory and visual hallucinations, paranoia	Emesis followed by charcoal and cathartic; patient may require sedation but usually can be talked down

Type	Clinical Assessment	Management
NITRATES OR NITRITES		
	Common cause of methemoglobinemia; initially asymptomatic cyanosis refractory to oxygen administration; tissue hypoxia develops as level increases, confusion, dizziness, tachycardia, dyspnea, coma, respiratory or cardiac arrest	Emesis or lavage followed b charcoal and cathartic; fo symptomatic patients or those with methemoglobi levels greater than 30%, administer tetramethylthionine chloride (methylene blue): 1 to 2 mg/kg of 1% solution IV over 5-10 min; if exposur is via topical route, remov clothing and wash skin wi water or saline using prot tive gloves and clothing
OPIATES		
	Lethargy or coma, pinpoint pupils, respiratory depression, pulmonary edema, hypotension	Lavage followed by charcoal and cathartic Naloxone (Narcan): a. Adult: 0.8 mg to 2 mg more IV push, repeat a necessary to reverse symptoms b. Pediatric: 0.8 mg to 2 IV push Naloxone may also be giv as continuous infusion: 1/ amp/hour

e	Clinical Assessment	Management
GANOPHOSPHATES		
	Increased salivation, diaphoresis, muscle weakness, bronchoconstriction, bradycardia, pulmonary edema, seizures, coma	Emesis or lavage followed by charcoal and cathartic; if exposure is via topical route, remove patient's clothing and wash skin with water or saline (NOTE: It is critical for all medical personnel to wear gloves and gown to handle patients and clothing since these poisons are readily absorbed through skin and mucous membranes and significant poisonings of health workers have occurred) 1. Atropine: a. Adult: 2-5 mg IV slowly b. Pediatric: 0.05 mg/kg IV; may repeat every 10-30 minutes 2. Pralidoxime (2-PAM) (Protopam chloride) given intravenously after atropine: a. Adult: 1 gm IV (500 mg/minute); may be repeated every 8-12 hours b. Pediatric: 25-50 mg/kg IV slowly; may be repeated every 8-12 hours

Type	Clinical Assessment	Management
PHENCYCLIDINE (PCP)		
	Confusion, agitation, nystagmus; visual, hearing, and perceptual disturbances; hypertension, tachycardia, psychosis, seizures, hyperthermia	Emesis or lavage followed b charcoal and cathartic; patient may require sedation; propranolol may be given for hypertension or tachycardia at 1 mg IV slowly; acid diuresis: asco bic acid 1-2 mg/L of IV fl to keep urine pH below
PHENOTHIAZINE		
	Anticholinergic symptoms (refer to p. 133, Anticholinergics); extrapyramidal signs: dyskinesia, dystonia, oculogyric and buccolingual crisis, parkinsonian symptoms	Emesis or lavage followed b charcoal and cathartic 1. Diphenhydramine (Be dryl): a. Adult: 25-50 mg IV IM b. Pediatric: 1 mg/kg up to 50 mg 2. Cogentin 1-2 mg IV (1 mg/minute)
SALICYLATE		
	Nausea, vomiting, tachypnea, hyperthermia, tinnitis, lethargy, seizures, metabolic acidosis	Emesis or lavage followed b charcoal and cathartic; obtain salicylate level 6 hours after ingestion; che electrolytes, anion gap; alkaline diuresis: sodium bicarbonate 1-2 mEq/kg dextrose 5% or dextrose 5% .25 normal saline; if p tient is dehydrated, infuse 10-15 ml/kg/hour, if not ml/kg/hour; perform exte nal cooling measures if pa tient is hyperthermic

ype	Clinical Assessment	Management
OLUENE		
	Toxicity occurs most frequently following repeated intentional inhalation; symptoms include dilated pupils, irritation of upper respiratory tract and lacrimation, headache, ataxia, muscle weakness, hematuria	Move patient to fresh air; lavage if large amount, cuffed endotracheal tube must be in place; use charcoal or cathartic; correct hypokalemia and acidosis with potassium and bicarbonate; monitor ABGs in symptomatic patients; (CAUTION: Hypocalcemia may ensue following fluid and electrolyte replenishment)
RICYCLIC ANTIDEPRESSANTS		
	Anticholinergic symptoms: disorientation, hallucinations, lethargy, coma, seizures, cardiac arrhythmias and conduction disturbances, respiratory depression; rapid progression	Lavage; charcoal and cathartic may be given repeatedly; closely monitor ECG 1. Phenytoin (Dilantin) can be given prophylactically or for treatment of seizures and cardiac conduction disturbances: a. Adult: 13-15 mg/kg IV b. Pediatric: 13-18 mg/kg IV, not to exceed 50 mg/minute; infuse in normal saline 2. Physostigmine may be given for anticholinergic symptoms (refer to p. 133, Anticholinergics); sodium bicarbonate 1-2 mEq/kg in IV solution if patient is acidotic or has arrhythmias refractory to above treatment 3. Lidocaine: a. Adult and pediatric: 1 mg/kg IV bolus, slowly for ventricular arrhythmias not responsive to above treatments

IMPLEMENTATION

I. Primary intervention
   A. Obtain patent airway
      1. Nasal pharyngeal airway
      2. Oral or nasal intubation if patient is obtunded
      3. Assisted ventilation if respiratory depression exists
      4. When patient is arousable enough to struggle with intubation b procedure is indicated, paralysis may be required: succinylcholi chloride—adults and pediatric: 1 mg/kg IV
   B. Manage circulation
      1. Obtain IV access with normal saline or lactated Ringer's solution
      2. Infuse TKO if patient is normotensive
      3. Give fluid challenge if systolic blood pressure less than 90 mm H
      4. If hypotension is unresponsive to fluid challenge, give
         a) Norepinephrine (Levophed): 4 mg in 250 ml dextrose 5%; titra to maintain systolic above 100 mm Hg
         b) Dopamine (Intropin): 200 to 800 mg in 250 ml dextrose 5 titrate to maintain systolic above 100 mm Hg
      5. Use cardiac monitor
      6. Insert indwelling urinary catheter to monitor output if patient is u conscious
   C. Administer medications
      1. Dextrose 50% of 25 gm and naloxone 0.8 mg to 2 mg IV push f lethargy or unresponsiveness
      2. Use specific antagonists and antidotes outlined in differential ma agement section
   D. Remove toxin
      1. Emesis
         a) Provide method of emptying gastric contents if patient able protect airway
         b) Give syrup of ipecac: adults: 30 ml; pediatric: 5 to 15 ml
         c) Give enough water to induce vomiting, usually 240 ml for adu or 120 to 180 ml for children who can ambulate
         d) Repeat ipecac in 20 to 30 minutes if emesis has not occurred stimulate the oropharynx to induce vomiting
         e) Emetic effect may persist for up to 6 hours; in most patients on 1 to 2 hours
         f) Benefits of gastric emptying are controversial; depending on tin since ingestion, some institutions elect to administer charco and cathartic initially rather than stimulating emesis

E. Prevent absorption
   1. Activated charcoal
      a) Absorbs substance not removed by emesis or lavage
      b) Dose: adult: 60-100 gm; pediatric: 30-60 gm
      c) Administer orally or through lavage tube
      d) Dose may be repeated when potentially toxic amounts of drugs have been ingested
   2. Cathartics
      a) Magnesium sulfate, sodium sulfate, or magnesium citrate: adult: 30 gm; pediatric: 250 mg/kg
      b) Administer orally or through lavage tube with or following charcoal
      c) Use caution in renal-impaired or congestive heart failure patients
F. Consider initiating Mental Health Hold (MHH) and need for restraints if patient wishes to leave department and is considered harm to self
G. Consider contacting regional poison center for consultation

. Secondary intervention

A. Obtain laboratory data
   1. Drug screens
      a) Quantitative levels useful for a few drugs such as alcohol, acetaminophen (should be drawn 4 hours or more after ingestion), antiepileptic drugs, salicylates (should be drawn 6 hours or more after ingestion)
      b) Qualitative screens may be useful if type of ingestion is unknown or when considering poisoning in unresponsive patient
      c) Patient should be treated according to clinical presentation, not solely by drug screen results (TREAT THE PATIENT—NOT THE POISON)
      d) Individual laboratories request blood or urine or both for specific screens
   2. Give electrolytes as outlined in differential management section
   3. Obtain ABGs if patient is obtunded, ventilated, or hypotensive
   4. Perform chest x-ray study after intubation or if aspiration is of concern
   5. Obtain 12-lead ECG if ingested drug is a cardiotoxin
B. Obtain serial vital signs and assessment of respiratory and mental status; patient's condition may deteriorate rapidly
C. Comfort patient after vomiting or lavage
D. Reassess circumstances of ingestion
   1. Accidental, suicidal, or recreational
   2. Identify precipitating event or circumstances
   3. Patient may deny suicidal gesture; confirm history with family or significant others whenever possible

4. Arrange psychiatric consultation for patients with suspected or co firmed intentional overdose

EVALUATION

I. Patient outcomes/criteria
   A. Vital signs within normal limits
   B. Evidence of pill fragments in emesis or lavage
   C. Appropriate mental status
   D. Resolution of presenting symptoms
   E. Agreement to psychiatric counseling if indicated
II. Document initial assessment, emergency department interventions, an patient's response to treatment
III. If previous patient outcomes are not reached, the emergency nurse shou reevaluate the interventions and change the plan of care accordingly

DISPOSITION

I. Admission criteria
   A. Patient requiring prolonged ventilatory assistance
   B. Ingestion of drugs causing various organ sequelae or those with pr longed duration
      1. Acids/alkalines
      2. Toxic acetaminophen
      3. Tricyclic antidepressants
      4. Cyanide
      5. Metals/iron
      6. Oral hypoglycemic agents
      7. Organophosphates
      8. Ingestion resulting in severe methemoglobinemia
   C. Patient still expressing suicidal thoughts requiring psychiatric admissio
II. Discharge guidelines
   A. Confirm psychiatric follow-up arrangements if appropriate
   B. Offer patient/family teaching
      1. Explain drug interactions such as alcohol and sedatives
      2. Give suggestions for keeping medications and chemicals away fro children to prevent accidental poisonings; advise family to kee syrup of ipecac at home
      3. Correct directions for taking prescribed medications when overdos was unintentional because of lack of knowledge
      4. Caution patient to expect black diarrheal stool as a result of charco and cathartic

CHAPTER 21

PSYCHIATRIC EMERGENCIES

IPLICATIONS FOR ACTION

behavioral crisis can occur in any setting. Assistance from the emergency epartment is often sought by family members, witnesses, or the patient. The nergent task is to protect the patient and others from harm, determine the use of the crisis, and initiate appropriate treatment and counseling. The posbility of metabolic abnormalities, toxins, or head trauma as causes for behavral crises must be considered.

In order to obtain a complete assessment of the situation, it is important to icit information from family and significant others since securing an accurate story from the patient may be difficult. For further information, refer to apendix B, "Crisis Intervention for Commonly Seen Behavioral Type Patients."

SSESSMENT

I. Initial observation
   A. Manner of presentation of patient's behavior
   B. Affect
II. Subjective assessment
   A. Patient's description of why he or she is seeking treatment
   B. Suicidal or homicidal thoughts
   C. Major life change or stress
   D. Past medical and psychiatric history, including medications
   E. Drug or alcohol use; overdose or recreational use
   F. Recent head trauma
   G. History of patient's behavior obtained from family, friends, police, or paramedics
   H. Hallucinations: auditory or visual
   I. Delusions or delirium
   J. Support systems

III. Objective assessment
   A. Vital signs
      1. Elevated temperature may be indicative of systemic illness
      2. Orthostatic vital signs needed if patient appears ataxic, dehydrat or poorly nourished
   B. Mental status, orientation, and appropriateness of conversation, me ory (refer to appendix B for complete mental status examination)
   C. Evidence of recent drug or alcohol ingestion: needle or track mar smell of alcohol on breath
   D. Affect or behavior indicating
      1. Depression
      2. Anxiety
      3. Rage
      4. Phobia
      5. Confusion or disorganization
      6. Paranoia
      7. Hallucinations
      8. Withdrawal

POTENTIAL NURSING DIAGNOSES/ANALYSIS

I. Anxiety
II. Communication, impaired: verbal
III. Coping, ineffective individual
IV. Grieving, anticipatory and dysfunctional
V. Health maintenance, alteration in
VI. Home maintenance management, impaired
VII. Injury: potential for poisoning and trauma
VIII. Knowledge deficit
IX. Mobility, impaired physical
X. Noncompliance
XI. Nutrition, alteration in: less than or more than body requirements
XII. Parenting, alteration in: actual or potential
XIII. Powerlessness
XIV. Rape trauma syndrome
XV. Self-care deficit: feeding, bathing/hygiene, dressing/grooming, toileti
XVI. Self-concept, disturbance in: body image, self-esteem, role performanc personal identity
XVII. Sensory-perceptual alteration: visual, auditory, kinesthetic
XVIII. Sleep pattern disturbance

XIX. Social isolation
XX. Spiritual distress (distress of the human spirit)
XXI. Thought processes, alteration in
XXII. Violence, potential for: self-directed or directed at others

PLANNING

I. Priorities for care
   A. Protection of patient and others from harm
   B. Ruling out medical or trauma cause for crisis
   C. Treating acute anxiety
II. Differential management

Types	Clinical Assessment	Management
FUNCTIONAL PSYCHOSIS		
	Clinical manifestations characterized by disturbances in perception, cognition, affect, and reality testing without an organic cause; most common presentations to the emergency department involve schizophrenia, manic-depressive illness, psychotic depression, and paranoia	Prevent patient from harming self or others; definitive diagnosis may not be obtainable while patient is in the emergency department; patients often require medication and psychiatric hospitalization with follow-up care; consider organic cause for behavior
ORGANIC ILLNESS		
	Physiological disturbance causing brain dysfunction, exhibited in behavior disorder manifested as altered mental status, disorientation, or decreased memory; can result from drug and alcohol use, toxic effects of prescribed or recreational drugs, withdrawal, overdose, medical illness, metabolic abnormalities, electrolyte imbalances, endocrine disorders, degenerative brain disease, infection, closed head injury	Obtain blood and urine drug screens, electrolytes, and glucose; perform medical workup indicated by suspected illness; obtain CT scans and skull x-ray studies as indicated

Types	Clinical Assessment	Management
SITUATIONAL RESPONSES		
	Behavior resulting from life change or major stress such as serious illness, loss of loved one, grief, change of job, victim of violence such as sexual assault, domestic violence, child abuse; patient may exhibit anxiety, depression, suicidal or homicidal thoughts	Prevent patient from harming s or others; assess need for immediate psychiatric interv tion; arrange counseling and social service support

IMPLEMENTATION

I. Primary intervention
   A. Protect the patient and staff from harm
      1. Employ restraints
         a) Use as safety measure, not discipline
         b) Apply as few restraints as possible
         c) Frequently check circulation of restrained patient
      2. Obtain Mental Health Hold (MHH)
         a) Indicated for suicidal, homicidal, or gravely disabled patient
         b) Patient may be placed by police, physician, or in certain state registered nurse
         c) Inform patient verbally and in writing
      3. Remove medications, sharp objects, and equipment from room
   B. Rule out organic cause for behavioral crisis
      1. Obtain laboratory data as indicated
         a) Drug toxicology screens, blood, and urine
         b) Complete blood count, electrolytes, glucose
      2. Assist with neurological evaluation

II. Secondary intervention
   A. Administer medications
      1. Medications for acute anxiety commonly given in emergency c partment (refer to table at end of care plan)
      2. Medications usually prescribed by psychiatrist
      3. Sedatives or tranquilizers

edications for Acute Anxiety*

pe	Recommended Dose	Considerations
NTIPSYCHOTICS		
aloperidol (aldol)	2.5-10 mg IM or IV (given at 2.5 mg/min IV route) (NOTE: IV usage is under research standard)	Most commonly used drug for agitated or violent patient; sedative response usually within minutes; complications include: hypotension, extrapyramidal symptoms; available in oral form
lorpromazine horazine)	25-50 mg IM	Dose for these antipsychotics very individual when given in oral form; complications include phenothiazine-induced extrapyramidal symptoms
uphenazine rolixin)	5-10 mg PO or IM	
iothixene avane)	5-10 mg IM	
ifluoperazine telazine)	1-5 mg IM	
ENZODIAZEPINES		
hlordiazepoxide ibrium)	50-100 mg IM or IV	Mix with accompanying diluent for IM use; dilute with saline or sterile water for IV use
iazepam alium)	2.5-10 mg IM, IV, or PO	Complications include respiratory depression, hypotension
orazepate ranxene)	7.5-30 mg PO	Not available in parenteral form

his list is not inclusive but represents the more common drugs used in the emergency partment.

4. Antipsychotic or psychotropic drugs
5. Antidepressants

B. Maintain consistent, calm approach
C. Provide environment with decreased stimulation for hallucinating, agitated, or combative patients
D. Offer fluids and bathroom privileges regularly
E. Note patient's intake and output

EVALUATION

I. Patient outcomes/criteria
   A. Vital signs within normal limits
   B. Decrease in presenting symptom behaviors
   C. Impulse control as evidenced by appropriate response to environme tal stimuli
   D. Ability to carry out activities of daily living
   E. Mental status more appropriate
II. Document initial assessment data, behavior changes, and responses communication efforts and medication; document rationale for restrain if used
III. If previous patient outcomes are not reached, the emergency nurse shou reevaluate the interventions and change the plan of care accordingly

DISPOSITION

I. Admission criteria
   A. Continued suicidal, homicidal, or violent behavior; patient unable care for self
   B. Further evaluation for psychiatric illness
   C. Drug therapy under controlled environment
II. Discharge guidelines
   A. Arrange outpatient counseling
   B. Give information concerning community resources (24-hour telephon crisis lines)
   C. Provide medication information

CHAPTER 22

RESPIRATORY DISTRESS

PLICATIONS FOR ACTION

way management is the prime consideration in acutely ill or injured pants and represents one of the greatest challenges and time-critical responilities in emergency medical treatment. As such, the patient in respiratory tress requires an immediate triage and assessment for potential lifesaving erventions. Once adequate oxygenation is assured, treatment of underlying thology becomes of concern.

The following protocol outlines the priorities for care of a patient in reiratory distress.

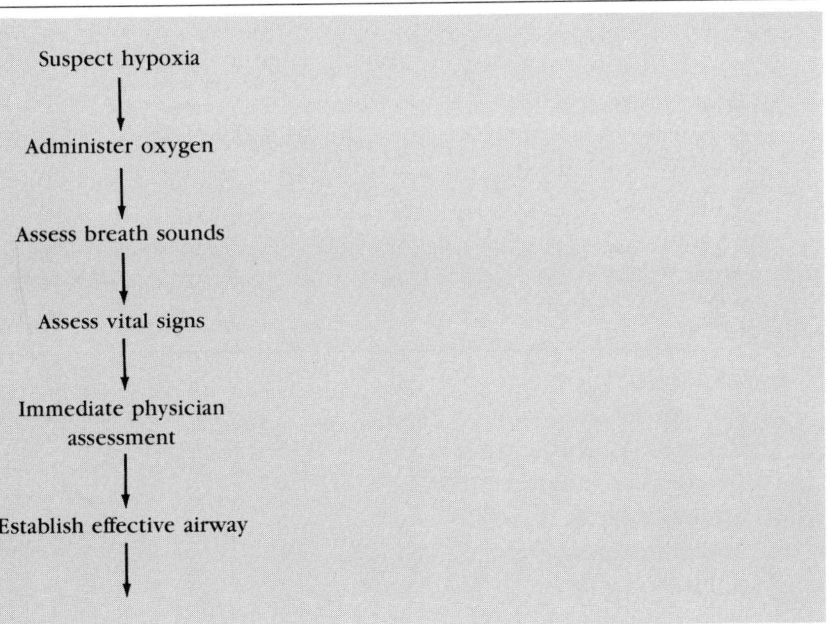

Continued.

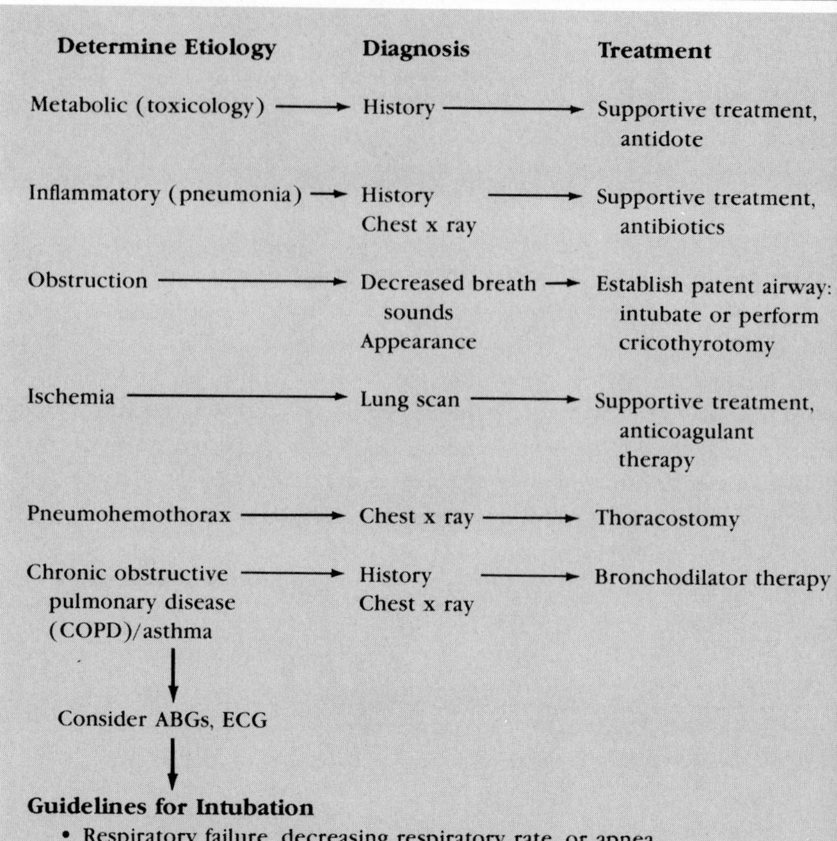

Determine Etiology
Diagnosis
Treatment
Metabolic (toxicology)
History
Supportive treatment, antidote
Inflammatory (pneumonia)
History
Chest x ray
Supportive treatment, antibiotics
Obstruction
Decreased breath sounds
Appearance
Establish patent airway: intubate or perform cricothyrotomy
Ischemia
Lung scan
Supportive treatment, anticoagulant therapy
Pneumohemothorax
Chest x ray
Thoracostomy
Chronic obstructive pulmonary disease (COPD)/asthma
History
Chest x ray
Bronchodilator therapy
Consider ABGs, ECG
Guidelines for Intubation
• Respiratory failure, decreasing respiratory rate, or apnea
• Po_2 <50 or Pco_2 >50
• Decreasing level of consciousness, fatigue
• Bradycardia in children

ASSESSMENT

I. Initial observation
   A. Skin color
   B. Respiratory effort
   C. Level of consciousness (LOC)
   D. Ability to speak
   E. Ability to cough
   F. Ability to move air
II. Subjective assessment
   A. History of present distress
      1. Onset of respiratory symptoms and activity before onset

2. Precipitating factors such as exposure to toxins, allergies, anxiety
3. Is patient becoming fatigued?
4. Reason for acute decompensation

B. Associated symptoms
1. Cough (describe sputum if produced)
2. Wheezing
3. Chest pain
   a) Pleuritic: pain with breathing
   b) Cardiac: substernal pain, any radiation of pain
4. Presence of orthopnea or paroxysmal nocturnal dyspnea (usually indicates cardiac origin)
5. Fever, chills
6. Ankle edema
7. Voice changes
8. Degree of anxiety

C. Measures taken to relieve symptoms, such as aspirin or acetaminophen, nebulizer, medications

D. Pertinent medical history
1. Lung or cardiac disease
2. Smoking history
3. Medications, including P.R.N. medications
4. Allergies
5. Hospitalizations, especially for respiratory disease
6. Any other previous illness
7. Trauma history

E. Recent stress, illness, or exertional activity (if trauma is the suspected cause of pain or respiratory distress, refer to Chapter 34, Care Plan for Major Multiple Trauma)

I. Objective assessment

A. Complete vital signs: note anything abnormal
1. Respiratory rate: greater than 18 to 20/min (40 to 60/min with children, refer to Chapter 19, Care Plan for Pediatric Emergencies for normal vital signs)
2. Pulse: tachycardia (bradycardia with children)
3. Blood pressure: note pulsus paradoxus, auscultate blood pressure (BP) at systolic level and note range where BP beats are changed in sound during inspiration (normal range = 10 to 12 mm Hg); abnormal range may be associated with congestive heart failure (CHF), pulmonary disease, cardiac tamponade
4. Temperature: may need rectal temperature if respiratory rate is increased

- B. Respiratory effort
  - 1. Physical examination
    - *a*) Skin color: cyanosis of lips and nailbeds or pallor
    - *b*) Breathing pattern, such as prolonged expiratory phase, use of accessory muscles
    - *c*) Stridor or audible wheezing
    - *d*) Tracheal deviation
    - *e*) Increased AP diameter (barrel chest)
  - 2. Breath sounds
    - *a*) Bilateral comparison
    - *b*) Presence or absence of rales, wheezes, rhonchi
    - *c*) Palpation (optional); note crepitus
- C. Neurological status
  - 1. Level of consciousness may be diminished because of hypoxia or more rarely hypercapnia
- D. Signs of external trauma
- E. Distended neck veins

POTENTIAL NURSING DIAGNOSES/ANALYSIS

- I. Airway clearance, ineffective
- II. Anxiety
- III. Breathing pattern, ineffective
- IV. Cardiac output, alteration in: decreased
- V. Comfort, alteration in: pain
- VI. Fear
- VII. Gas exchange, impaired
- VIII. Tissue perfusion, alteration in: cerebral, cardiopulmonary

PLANNING

- I. Priorities for care
  - A. Establishment and maintenance of patent airway
  - B. Isolation of cause of respiratory distress; initiation of treatment
  - C. Relieving patient's anxiety
  - D. Immediate physician assessment
  - E. Preparation for active airway management
- II. Differential management

pe of Distress	Clinical Assessment	Management
ULMONARY		
sthma	Reversible, episodic constriction of bronchial smooth muscle from hyperactive airways, excess mucous production, mucosal edema; associated symptoms include bilateral wheezing, tachypnea, tachycardia, air hunger, use of accessory muscles	Obtain intravenous access, administer oxygen 3-6 L/min via nasal prongs, use bronchodilators, perform cardiac monitoring, provide reassurance, obtain theophylline level if patient takes medication; obtain complete blood count if patient is febrile
nronic Obstruc-ve Pulmonary isease (COPD)	Chronic, irreversible obstructive disease of the airway, accompanied by reversible bronchospasms; frequently associated with prolonged expiratory phase, barrel chest, distant breath sounds, signs of right heart failure	Administer low-flow oxygen less than 3 L/min via nasal prongs or Venturi mask at 25%, perform cardiac monitoring; use bronchodilators; obtain theophylline level if patient takes medicine; obtain complete blood count if patient is febrile
neumonia	Fever, cough, chills, chest pain; often preceded by recent upper respiratory tract illness; may hear rales, rhonchi	Administer oxygen at 2-4 L/min via nasal prongs; obtain complete blood count, sputum cultures, chest x-ray study; patient may require hospital admission for intravenous antibiotics
ılmonary mbolus	Pleuritic chest pain, tachypnea, dyspnea, tachycardia, cough with hemoptysis, cyanosis, diaphoresis, anxiety; high incidence in patients with history of immobilization, phlebitis, deep vein thrombosis, long-bone fracture, or oral contraceptive use	Institute cardiac monitoring; obtain intravenous access; obtain chest x-ray study; obtain arterial blood gases; diagnose with lung scan or angiography; treat with anticoagulants; obtain baseline PT/PTT; administer heparin 5-10 units IV bolus, follow with continuous infusion drip; analgesia usually requires hospital admission

Type of Distress	Clinical Assessment	Management
Croup	Seen in children ages 6 months-3 years; usually with signs/symptoms of upper respiratory infection preceding; child usually looks well, becomes worse at night with stridor and characteristic barking cough; child may improve when taken out in cool night air; will drink fluids; tachypnea with accessory muscle use; child may be febrile	Provide cool oxygen or room air mist, PO or IV hydration if necessary; obtain chest x-ray study (will be normal); obtain laboratory data complete blood count-WBC (nonspecific) blood cultures negative; administer medications: Vaponephrin (racemic epinephrine); if used, child will need to be admitted because of rebound effect with worse symptoms; steroids remain controversial
Bronchiolitis	Seen in children ages <2 years with peak incidence in <6 months; child usually has preceding upper respiratory infection, appears well but is tachypenic, wheezing, with accessory muscle use; 90% of all cases are caused by respiratory syncytial virus (RSV)	Administer humidified oxygen given fluid replacement IV and/or PO; prepare to intubate if there is apnea or decreased respiratory rate with brachycardia; administer medications: epinephrine 0.01 mg/kg (not to exceed 0.3 ml) S.Q. (under 6 months, patient will not respond well because of scarcity of bronchiole smooth muscle); administer bronchodilators
Hyperventilation Syndrome	Rapid, shallow breathing resulting in respiratory alkalosis, circumoral and peripheral paresthesias, carpopedal spasm; may be caused by anxiety or response to underlying disorder such as compensation for acidosis, fever, pulmonary, or neurological disorder, hypovolemia	If anxiety is cause, use calm approach to get patient to rebreathe into small paper bag or use nonrebreather mask; treat underlying pathology if present

e of Distress	Clinical Assessment	Management
STRUCTED AIRWAY		
	Sudden history of choking on food; foreign body is observed; if patient is conscious, may be clutching throat, unable to speak, dusky and cyanotic, with coughing, wheezing, upper respiratory infection history with sudden audible stridor and inability to handle secretions	Remove foreign body; mobilize for intubation or cricothyrotomy (refer to appendix A for procedure and equipment); specific management depends on etiology
EUMOTHORAX		
	Sudden chest pain that increases with deep inspiration; decreased or absent breath sounds on affected side; asymmetrical chest wall movement; dyspnea	Administer oxygen 3-5 L/min via nasal prongs, obtain intravenous access; prepare for thoracostomy (refer to appendix A for procedure and equipment); administer pain medications as necessary
RITONSILLAR ABSCESS		
	Frequently occurs as the end point of upper respiratory infection with fever, malaise, voice changes, and difficulty in swallowing; tonsillar tissue potentially could occlude the airway; drooling is suggestive of acute upper airway obstruction	Visualize tonsils, maintain airway; often incision and drainage on an inpatient or outpatient basis are needed; administer antibiotic therapy
AUMA-RELATED RESPIRATORY DISTRESS		
	(Refer to Chapter 34, Care Plan for Major Multiple Trauma)	

Type of Distress	Clinical Assessment	Management
EPIGLOTTITIS		
	Usually seen in children ages 3-7 years; abrupt onset with potential for obstructed airway and arrest; child looks very sick: poor color, tachypneic, cyanotic, sits erect with head in sniffing position, drools and will not take fluids; may have stridor but no barking cough; usually febrile	Airway management is priority: prepare to intubate or perform cricothyrotomy (refer to appendix A for procedure and equipment); administer 100% humidified oxygen by mask; obtain intravenous access; supportive treatment includes: ampicillin 100-200 mg/kg q4h and chloramphenicol 75-100 mg/kg q6h or moxalactam 150 mg/kg q8h; obtain blood cultures (will be positive for hemophilus influenza; WBC will show left shift); chest x-ray study will show enlarged epiglottis; do not attempt to visualize epiglottis unless prepared to intubate or attempt may cause upper edema or laryngospasm; intubation in operating room is preferred
HYPOXIA WITH CHEST PAIN		
	(Refer to Chapter 4, Care Plan for Chest Pain)	

IMPLEMENTATION

I. Primary intervention
   A. Manage airway
      1. Oxygenate
         a) Nasal cannula can deliver FIO_2 of 24% to 44% with 2 to 6 L/min
         b) O_2 mask can deliver 40% to 60% O_2 with 6 to 10 L/min
         c) Nonrebreathing mask can deliver 60% to 100% with 8 to 1[illegible] L/min

2. Intubate for
   a) Respiratory arrest or severe grade apnea or respiratory failure: Po_2 <50 $P\dot{c}o_2$ >50; decreased level of consciousness; bradycardia with children
   b) Prepare the following equipment
      (1) Laryngoscope and blades
      (2) Cuffed endotracheal tubes
      (3) Magill forceps (for nasotracheal route)
      (4) Stylet
      (5) 10-ml syringe
      (6) Water-soluble lubricant
      (7) Oxygen reservoir bag and mask
      (8) Suction
   c) Medications needed on hand
      (1) Lidocaine: 1.5 mg/kg
      (2) Atropine: 0.5 mg
      (3) Succinylcholine: 1.5 mg/kg
      (4) Pavolon: 0.1 mg/kg
   d) Check endotracheal tube placement by auscultating breath sounds bilaterally in both axillae; observe for equal chest expansion; feel for warm exhalations at endotracheal tube opening; obtain chest x-ray study for exact placement; secure tube in place
   e) Possible complications: broken teeth, vocal cord damage, tracheal injury, improper tube placement, aspiration
   f) Restrain and reassure patient as necessary

B. Obtain intravenous access
   1. Dextrose 5% at TKO rate as access for medications (for uncomplicated asthma, airway obstruction)
   2. Dextrose 5% 0.45 normal saline at 125 to 150 ml/hr for rehydration (for asthma, COPD, pulmonary embolism)
   3. 0.9 normal saline at variable rate if patient is at risk for developing hypotension or life-threatening complications (hemopneumothorax)

C. Perform laboratory tests
   1. Theophylline level (ordered if patient takes medication) to determine if patient is in therapeutic range
   2. Complete blood count if patient is febrile or history suggests upper respiratory infection (URI)
   3. Electrolytes as baseline data for hospital admission if appropriate for institution

4. Arterial blood gases if patient is acutely decompensated or intubat (REMINDER: P_{CO_2} will be elevated as chronic state in patients w COPD)

D. Monitor cardiac activity
   1. Hypoxia may cause dysrhythmia; patient may frequently be tach cardic, except children who usually become bradycardic w hypoxia
   2. Obtain 12-lead ECG

E. Obtain chest x-ray study to rule out infiltrates, pneumonia, pneum thorax, air trapping

F. Administer medications
   1. Bronchodilators
      a) Metaproterenol (Alupent): 0.3 to 0.5 ml 5% solution in 2.5- normal saline given nebulized every 1 to 2 hours; used as need until signs of toxicity occur (heart rate >150)
      b) Isoetharine (Bronchosol): 0.5 ml of 1% solution diluted in 1.5 normal saline given nebulized every 2 to 4 hours; side effec increased heart rate, dysrhythmias; use carefully if underlyi heart disease present, patient hypoxic, or has heart rate >13
      c) Aminophylline: 5 to 7 mg/kg loading dose, 0.4 to 0.2 mg/ 1-hour maintenance dose; decrease dosage in patients with co gestive heart failure, those who smoke or have liver disease; gi maintenance dose while awaiting blood levels; side effects inclu tachycardia, headache, nausea, vomiting, diarrhea, convulsion
      d) Epinephrine: 0.2 to 0.5 ml subcutaneously × 3 every 30 to minutes as needed; side effects: tachycardia, elevated blood pre sure, arrhythmias
      e) Terbutaline: 0.25 mg subcutaneously; may repeat × 1 if no r sponse in 30 minutes; do not use if patient >40 years of age has a history of ischemic heart disease
      f) Vaponephrin (racemic epinephrine): 0.5 ml of a 2% solution luted in 2.5 ml sterile H_2O given nebulized; if this medication used, children must be admitted because of rebound effect wh drug wears off (after 4 hours)
   2. Others
      a) Steroids: Solu-Medrol 60 to 250 mg every 6 hours; may take 3 6 hours for decreased mucosal edema; restores responsivene to adrenergic bronchodilators; side effects: hypokalemia mas signs of infection, especially fever, increases incidence of pept ulcer especially in COPD patient; pediatric dose: 0.25 to 0 mg/kg/dose every 6 hours using dexamethasone (Decadron)

b) Antibiotics: for infection according to physician's instructions
G. Follow guidelines as indicated in differential management section
Secondary intervention
A. Perform chest physiotherapy (clapping and postural drainage)
B. Suction endotrachea as necessary
C. Position head of bed for patient's comfort and ease of breathing
D. Administer oral fluids and humidified oxygen
E. Obtain serial vital signs
F. Perform continuous cardiac monitoring
G. Give explanations to patient and family to diminish anxiety

VALUATION

I. Patient outcomes/criteria
A. Respiratory status improvement: good color, comfortable respiratory rate, clear and equal breath sounds (or return to baseline with asthma patient); patient handles own secretions well
B. Normal heart rate
C. Diminished or absent wheezes
D. Normal pulsus paradoxus (10 to 12 mm Hg)
E. Diminished anxiety
I. Document initial assessment data, emergency department intervention, and patient's response to treatment
I. If previous patient outcomes are not reached, the emergency nurse should reevaluate the interventions and change the plan of care accordingly

ISPOSITION

Admission criteria
A. Unresolved respiratory distress
B. Patient who is intubated
C. Pulmonary embolus, pneumonia, pneumothorax, or conditions requiring IV antibiotics
D. History of return visits (three in 48 hours) to emergency department for therapy
E. Spirometrics: FeVI <800 ml
Discharge guidelines
A. Give instructions concerning disease process
B. Offer instructions on follow-up activity, clinics, private physician, etc.
C. Instruct patient on medications
D. Instruct patient and parents with sick child, including when to return to hospital

CHAPTER 23

SEIZURES

IMPLICATIONS FOR ACTION

The patient who arrives in the emergency department actively having a seizur requires immediate attention. Intervention is directed toward maintenance c airway, protection from injury, and ending the seizure activity. The primar interventions are carried out before obtaining a thorough history and physica assessment. Patients arriving in the department in a postictal state may presen a confusing picture unless there is a witness to the seizure. Other etiologies c altered mental status or unresponsiveness must be considered if the cause c seizure activity is not known.

ASSESSMENT

- I. Initial observation
  - A. Current seizure activity (focal, generalized, or both)
  - B. Respiratory status
  - C. Level of consciousness
  - D. Skin color
- II. Subjective assessment
  - A. Past medical history
    1. Seizure history
    2. Recent illness or trauma
    3. Drug or alcohol abuse
  - B. Prescribed medication and compliance
  - C. History of aura
  - D. Witnesses' accounts of event
- III. Objective assessment
  - A. Vital signs
    1. Expect abnormality in pulse and blood pressure and watch for re turn to normal parameters
    2. Note temperature; may indicate infection as cause for seizure
  - B. Description of seizure if witnessed in emergency department
    1. Preseizure activity

   2. Duration of seizure
   3. Type and progression of movement, extremities involved
   4. Incontinence
   5. Response to treatment if given
   6. Status epilepticus: seizure activity lasting greater than 3 minutes or when patient remains unresponsive between seizures

C. Length of postictal period and improvement of mental status over time
   1. If in status epilepticus, patient will not become alert between seizures
   2. If patient's mental status remains depressed after seizures have been controlled, consider other pathology

D. Concurrent injuries
   1. Lacerations of tongue or oral mucosa; loose or broken teeth
   2. Abrasions or lacerations suffered when patient falls to ground or during seizure
   3. Skeletal injuries: cervical spine, skull, or other bones; shoulder dislocations and thoracic or lumbar vertebrae injuries are common

E. Incontinence

F. Presence of emesis

G. Oral trauma

SSIBLE NURSING DIAGNOSES/ANALYSIS

. Airway clearance, ineffective
. Breathing patterns, ineffective
. Communication, impaired: verbal
. Injury: trauma, potential for
. Knowledge deficit (of medications)
. Noncompliance (with medications)

ANNING

Priorities for care

A. During seizure
   1. Protecting airway
   2. Preventing injury to patient
   3. Stopping seizure activity

B. After seizure
   1. Evaluating cause of seizure
   2. Completing medical and neurological evaluation for first seizure
   3. Monitoring vital signs and mental status

Differential management

Seizure Etiology	Clinical Assessment	Management
FIRST ADULT SEIZURE		
	Generally caused by infection, trauma, alcoholism, a space-occupying lesion (tumor or hematoma), metabolic abnormality, or is drug induced; focal seizures suggest a structural lesion	Patient is usually admitted for complete neurological workup; perform laboratory tests, EEG, CT scan
KNOWN SEIZURE DISORDER		
	Etiology may be idiopathic epilepsy, posttrauma, post-craniotomy, or related to alcohol use; often associated with medication noncompliance	Perform specific antiepileptic drug screen; administer additional medication for subtherapeutic levels (refer to medication table in this care plan, p. 164)
ALCOHOL WITHDRAWAL SEIZURE		
	Normally occurs 24-72 hours after cessation of alcohol; patients rarely have focal or status seizures	Usually not treated with anticonvulsants (refer to Chapter 3, Care Plan for Alcohol Withdrawal)
HYPOGLYCEMIC SEIZURE		
	Suspect in patient with history of diabetes; alcoholic patients are also frequently hypoglycemic	Rapid improvement in mental status with dextrose 50% 25 gm IV bolus
FEBRILE SEIZURE		
	Most common cause of seizure in children 6 months to 3 years; associated with rapid increase in temperature rather than any specific temperature level; seizure is usually of short duration with a short postictal phase	Isolate source of fever (refer to Chapter 19, Care Plan for Pediatric Emergencies)

MPLEMENTATION

I. Primary intervention
  A. Patient who is having a seizure
    1. Insert oral or nasopharyngeal airway or bite block (padded tongue blade) before jaws clench; do not force to avoid dental or soft tissue injury
    2. Assist patient to bed or floor, provide protective environment, protect extremities but do not forcibly restrain
    3. Administer oxygen via nasal cannula
    4. Suction as necessary and place patient in lateral position to prevent aspiration
  B. Status epilepticus
    1. Provide care as previously outlined, but patient will require intubation
    2. Insert IV for circulatory access
  C. Administer medications (refer to table in this section)
    1. Diazepam is given initially
    2. Phenobarbital and phenytoin in loading doses calculated by weight
    3. Dextrose 50% IV bolus to reverse hypoglycemia; naloxone hydrochloride (Narcan) to rule out drug intoxication as cause of seizure
    4. Thiamine 100 mg slow IV; given with dextrose 50% to prevent Wernicke's encephalopathy in malnourished alcoholic patients

II. Secondary intervention
  A. After seizure
    1. Maintain lateral position
    2. Evaluate vital signs and neurological status q15 minutes until patient is stable
  B. Obtain laboratory data
    1. Specific drug levels if patient is on antiepileptic medications
    2. If etiology of seizure is unknown, patient will require Narcan, electrolytes, glucose or dextrostix, toxicology screens, blood cultures, skull x-ray studies, CT scan, lumbar puncture
  C. Provide emotional support to patient and family

II. Medications

Type	Recommended Dose	Indications for Use	Considerations
DIAZEPAM (VALIUM)			
	1. Adult: 5-15 mg IV (not to exceed 5 mg/min) 2. Pediatric: 0.1-0.3 mg/kg (0.5-2 mg/min)	To halt seizure activity	Half-life is 7 minutes; complications includ hypotension and respiratory depression
PHENYTOIN			
	1. Adult: 13-15 mg/kg for IV load 2. Pediatric: 13-18 mg/kg for IV load	Stabilizes seizure threshold and depresses seizure activity	Dilute in normal saline it precipitates with dextrose, e.g.: 1 gm Dilantin in 100 ml normal saline over 2 minutes or longer; half-life is 7-48 hours (average 48); IV dos peaks in 15 minutes; oral dose peaks in 4- hours; complications include respiratory d pression, hypotensio bradydysrhythmias, pain at IV site
PHENOBARBITAL			
	1. Adult: 30-130 mg IV over 5-10 min (may repeat every 10-15 min until seizures are controlled—up to 1 gm) 2. Pediatric: 10-20 mg/kg IV or 6-10 mg/kg IM	For status epilepticus	Complications include: respiratory depressio hypotension; respiratory depression mor common if given wit diazepam

VALUATION

I. Patient outcomes/criteria
   A. Return to normal mentation
   B. No further seizure activity
I. Document initial assessment data, emergency interventions, and the patient's response to treatment
I. If previous patient outcomes are not reached, the emergency nurse should reevaluate the interventions and change the plan of care accordingly

ISPOSITION

. Admission criteria
   A. Usually only for first seizure
   B. Status epilepticus
. Discharge guidelines
   A. Instruct patient and family regarding cause of seizure and care to be given if patient has seizure at home
   B. Emphasize medication compliance and follow-up care
   C. Instruct patient and family in state law restrictions on patient's driving for a specific length of time after seizure activity

CHAPTER 24

SICKLE CELL CRISIS

IMPLICATIONS FOR ACTION

Most patients entering the emergency department in sickle cell crisis ha been previously diagnosed with the disorder. It is important, however, to ev uate the patient during each visit for possible complications of the disea Multiple small thromboses and infarctions in the microcirculatory system c cause variable symptomatology, ranging from decreased mental status to loc ized or generalized pain.

Patient education is vital because of the chronic nature of the disea Information regarding adequate hydration and nutrition, susceptibility to fection, and potential for narcotic addiction needs to be included with d charge instructions.

ASSESSMENT

I. Initial observation
   A. Crying or writhing in pain
   B. Disease found primarily in Blacks
II. Subjective assessment
   A. Past medical history
      1. Patient usually diagnosed during infancy but not seen until about months of age
      2. Frequency and length of crises
      3. Precipitating factors include illness, dehydration, strenuous ex cise, emotional stress, exposure to high altitude, cold, or pregnanc
      4. Patients may have narcotic addiction related to chronic use for pa
   B. Characteristics of crisis
      1. Location and severity of pain: usually in joints, chest, back, or abd men
      2. Dyspnea
      3. Weakness and fatigue
III. Objective assessment
   A. Vital signs

1. Tachycardia and tachypnea are common
2. Patient is febrile if infection precipitated crisis

B. Mental status

C. Clinical signs of dehydration
1. Dry skin and mucous membranes
2. Decreased skin turgor

D. Patient may be pale or jaundiced

E. Possible swollen joints

F. Hematuria

G. Check peripheral pulses (extensive sickling causes vascular compromise)

)SSIBLE NURSING DIAGNOSES/ANALYSIS

I. Anxiety

I. Comfort, alteration in: pain

I. Coping, ineffective family: compromised

/. Fluid volume deficit, actual or potential

'. Gas exchange, impaired

I. Knowledge deficit (of disease process)

I. Tissue perfusion, alteration in: cerebral, cardiopulmonary, renal, gastrointestinal, peripheral

.ANNING

. Priorities for care
  A. Oxygenation
  B. Intravenous hydration
  C. Alleviation of pain

. Pathophysiology
  A. Sickle cell disease is genetically transmitted and is characterized by abnormal hemoglobin and fragile erythrocytes, which cause a hemolytic anemia and sludging in the capillaries
  B. Associated complications of sickle cell anemia and crisis
    1. Abdominal pain resembling an acute abdominal condition
    2. Lesions in the central nervous system (cerebral thrombosis)
    3. Renal failure; decreased ability to concentrate urine
    4. Cardiac arrhythmias, especially atrial; congestive heart failure
    5. Vascular occlusion to any site
    6. Greater potential for infection
    7. Decreased life span

Differential management

Types of Crises	Clinical Assessment	Management
PAINFUL (MOST COMMON)		
	Blood flow is reduced or blocked to tissues and organs; pain frequently has onset in morning occurring in back, joints, and extremities; abdominal pain may be present; there is hematuria and elevated temperature	Obtain intravenous access, perform hydration, administer nasal oxygen 2-4 L/min; analgesia; recommend bed r
APLASTIC		
	Most common cause is infection; increase in pallor or more lethargy than usual	Reticulocyte count will determine; in addition to interven tions mentioned above, pack red cells; transfusion determined on individual basis
SEQUESTRATION (PRIMARILY SEEN IN CHILDREN)		
	Massive splenomegaly; anemia; sudden onset of nausea, vomiting, rigid abdomen; hypovolemic shock occurs most commonly between 6 months and 6 years; may be precipitated by infection	Obtain intravenous access, perform fluid resuscitation with lactated Ringer's; possible su gical intervention for recurr crisis

IMPLEMENTATION

I. Primary intervention
  A. Administer oxygen via nasal prongs at 2 to 6 L/min
  B. Perform intravenous hydration with normal saline or dextrose 5% half normal saline; infuse rapidly, at least 250 ml/hour; observe for c gestive failure if patient is over 30 years old
  C. Monitor cardiac activity to evaluate dysrhythmias
  D. Administer analgesia
    1. Narcotic analgesia is normally required to abate pain, frequer meperidine (Demerol) 50 to 125 mg plus hydroxyzine 20 to 75 initially, then q3h twice intramuscularly or IV
    2. Prolonged use of meperidine should be avoided because of risk seizures in children; instead use

a) Codeine: 3 mg/kg
b) Morphine: 0.1 mg to 0.2 mg/kg q1-4h

E. Obtain laboratory data
1. Complete blood count to rule out infection and possible sepsis
2. Sickle cell screening if condition is not previously diagnosed
3. Electrolytes to rule out acidosis
4. Arterial blood gases if hypoxia is of concern

F. Monitor intake and output

Secondary intervention

A. Provide comfort
1. Local heat to affected areas
2. Rest

B. Educate family and patient and provide counseling

'ALUATION

. Patient outcomes/criteria

A. Relief of pain evidenced by
1. Patient's subjective behavior: patient able to rest or sleep, not crying or moaning
2. Fewer requests for pain medication

B. Vital signs within normal limits

. Document initial assessment data, emergency department interventions, and patient's response to treatment

. If previous patient outcomes are not reached, the emergency nurse should reevaluate the interventions and change the plan of care accordingly

ISPOSITION

Admission criteria

A. Inability to relieve symptoms or hypoxia

B. Sequestration of spleen

C. Associated complications that warrant admission, such as stroke, pulmonary infarction, prolonged priapism

Discharge guidelines

A. Provide discharge instructions
1. Use of analgesics
2. Oral hydration
3. Continued rest
4. Returning if symptoms recur
5. Seeking prompt medical treatment when ill

B. Document instructions and medications given

C. Give psychosocial counseling as indicated

CHAPTER 25

SYNCOPE

IMPLICATIONS FOR ACTION

Syncope is a frightening experience for the patient as well as for witnes
Although the majority of syncopal episodes are the result of vasovagal eve
various neurological, cardiovascular, or metabolic abnormalities can resul
temporary loss of consciousness. Interventions are aimed at excluding th
abnormalities as causes. Because the event is often not observed, a thoro
history and assessment are essential. The following protocol outlines the
orities for care in the patient who has syncope.

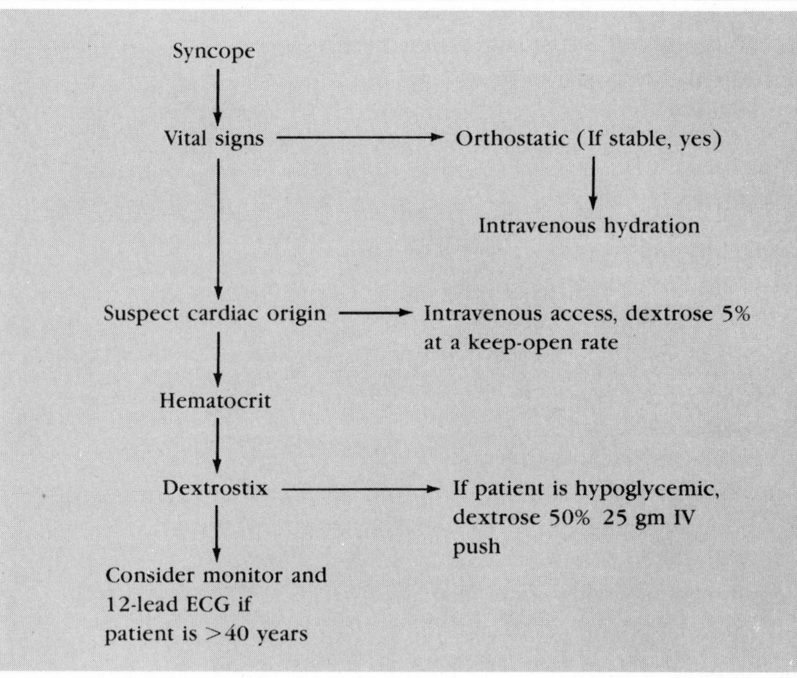

.SSESSMENT

I. Initial observation
   A. Skin color
   B. Respiratory effort
   C. Level of consciousness
:I. Subjective assessment
   A. Description of episode
      1. Sequence of preceding events
      2. Duration of episode
      3. Total or near loss of consciousness
      4. Actions that relieve symptoms such as lying down, sitting, eating
   B. Associated symptoms
      1. Nausea, vomiting, diarrhea (hematemesis, melena)
      2. Headache, dizziness, vertigo
      3. Dyspnea, chest pain, palpitations
      4. Chills, diaphoresis
   C. Time of last meal
   D. Past medical history
      1. Head trauma
      2. Known cardiac disease, dysrhythmias, diabetes, seizure disorder
      3. Medications and allergies
I. Objective assessment
   A. Complete vital signs with orthostatics
   B. Mental status
   C. Checking mucous membranes and skin turgor for hydration status
   D. Gynecological history for women
      1. Date and description of last menstrual period
      2. Gravity and parity
      3. Vaginal bleeding

OSSIBLE NURSING DIAGNOSES/ANALYSIS

I. Airway clearance, ineffective
II. Anxiety
III. Breathing pattern, ineffective
IV. Cardiac output, alteration in: decreased
V. Fluid volume deficit, actual
VI. Gas exchange, impaired
VII. Nutrition, alteration in: less than body requirements
III. Tissue perfusion, alteration in: cerebral, cardiopulmonary

PLANNING

I. Priorities for care
   A. Hemodynamic stabilization
   B. Isolating cause of syncopal episode
II. Differential management

Type	Clinical Assessment (Causes)	Management
CARDIOVASCULAR		
	Dysrhythmias, valvular heart disease, or pulmonary embolus may result in chest pain, diaphoresis, pallor, or cyanosis; dehydration may result from vomiting, diarrhea, gastrointestinal bleeding, ruptured ectopic pregnancy; vasovagal episode can be caused by overstimulation of parasympathetic nervous system resulting in bradycardia, hypotension, and weakness; autonomic dysfunction also may result in syncope	12-lead ECG; treat dysrhythmias as indicated (refer to Chapter 17, Care Plan for Medical Cardiopulmonary Arrest); obtain a lung scan; attach Holter monitor, arrange bundle of His studies; administer intravenous hydration; if possible, identify and avoid precipitating cause
NEUROGENIC		
	Altered mental status, hypertension, abnormal breathing patterns; focal neurological signs may indicate head trauma, cerebral vascular accident, hypertensive encephalopathy, or epilepsy	Perform serial mental status assessment; neurological examination by physician may require CT scan or EEG (refer to Chapter 27, Care Plan for Unresponsive Patient)
METABOLIC		
	Hypoglycemia indicated by hunger, diaphoresis, weakness, headache; anemia; hypoxia, hypercarbia, hyperventilation, and drug reaction may also cause syncope	Dextrostix blood; if abnormal, send serum glucose; dextrose 50% IV push if indicated; obtain hematocrit; manage airway

IMPLEMENTATION

I. Primary intervention
   A. Obtain intravenous access if indicated by assessment
      1. Administer dextrose 5% TKO if suspected cardiac etiology
      2. Use normal saline or lactated Ringer's solution if patient is orthostatic
      3. Administer dextrose 50% one amp and Naloxone 0.8 to 2 mg intravenously for depressed mental status
   B. Administer oxygen 3 to 6 L/min via nasal prongs if patient is exhibiting respiratory distress
   C. Perform diagnostic studies
      1. Hematocrit
      2. Dextrostix; serum glucose if abnormal
      3. Bedside cardiac monitoring and 12-lead ECG
      4. Arterial blood gases to assess oxygenation if patient is cyanotic or has depressed respiratory effort or distress

II. Secondary intervention
   A. Obtain serial vital signs and mental status assessments
   B. Provide nourishment if hypoglycemia is determined as cause of syncope
   C. Inform patient and family of emergency department course
   D. Provide comfort measures and reassurance

EVALUATION

I. Patient outcomes/criteria
   A. Return to normal mental status
   B. Resolution of orthostatic vital signs
   C. Dysrhythmia stabilization
   D. Serum glucose within normal limits
   E. Blood loss stabilized
   F. Absence of respiratory distress

II. Document initial assessment data, emergency department interventions, and patient's response to treatment

III. If previous patient outcomes are not reached, the emergency nurse should reevaluate the interventions and change the plan of care accordingly

DISPOSITION

I. Admission criteria
   A. Patients with dysrhythmias or cardiac disease
   B. Intracranial event

   C. Continuing blood loss such as with gastrointestinal bleeding or ruptured ectopic pregnancy

II. Discharge guidelines
   A. Instruct patient to avoid precipitating cause, if known
   B. Provide family education concerning immediate treatment of person with syncopal episode
      1. Assist person to reclining position
      2. Do not force food or fluids if person is unconscious
   C. Instruct patient to return to emergency department if episode recurs
   D. Arrange follow-up if further diagnostic studies are indicated

CHAPTER 26

SYSTEMIC ALLERGIC REACTION

IPLICATIONS FOR ACTION

a allergic reaction can range from mild symptoms to total respiratory and rculatory collapse. Careful and continuous assessment of the patient is vital. nticipation of potential complications will lead to a smooth resuscitation.

SSESSMENT

I. Initial observation
   A. Respiratory effort
   B. Skin color
   C. Presence of edema
I. Subjective assessment
   A. Presenting symptoms
      1. Dyspnea, tightness in chest
      2. Difficulty swallowing
      3. Sensation of swollen lips, tongue, or fingers
      4. Weakness, dizziness, syncope
      5. Anxiety, feeling of suffocation
   B. Associated history
      1. Time of onset of symptoms
      2. Sensitizing agent, if known
      3. Allergies; history of similar reactions
      4. Underlying respiratory problems
I. Objective assessment
   A. Vital signs, especially respiratory rate
   B. Respiratory status: observe for coughing, wheezing, or stridor; change or loss of voice or swelling of mucous membranes; shortness of breath
   C. Mental status: restlessness or agitation

- D. Skin condition
  1. Diaphoresis
  2. Warmth
  3. Rash or wheals (hives)
  4. Flushing, localized tenderness
  5. Edema
- E. Hypotension

POSSIBLE NURSING DIAGNOSES/ANALYSIS

- I. Airway clearance, ineffective
- II. Anxiety
- III. Breathing pattern, ineffective
- IV. Cardiac output, alteration in: decreased
- V. Fluid volume deficit, potential
- VI. Gas exchange, impaired
- VII. Tissue perfusion, alteration in: cerebral, cardiopulmonary

PLANNING

- I. Priorities for care
  - A. Treat respiratory compromise and hypotension
  - B. Alleviate other signs of allergic reaction

IMPLEMENTATION

- I. Primary intervention
  - A. Treat anaphylactic shock
    1. Maintain airway; prepare to intubate; cricothyrotomy may be r quired if laryngeal edema prevents intubation
    2. Administer oxygen at 2 to 6 L/min
    3. Obtain intravenous access; normal saline for hypotension
    4. May need to use pneumatic antishock trousers
    5. Administer medications: IV route if patient is in shock (refer to box in Chapter 17, pp. 113-115, for dosages)
       - *a*) Epinephrine (1:10,000 dilution) at usual dosage of 1 ml 1:10,000 solution, repeat q5 min as necessary
       - *b*) Vasopressors: Norepinephrine (Levophed)
Metaraminol (Aramine)
Dopamine (Intropin)

c) Steroids: hydrocortisone (Solu-Cortef)
d) Bronchodilators: aminophylline at usual dosage of 250 to 500 mg initially, then 0.5 mg/kg/hr
e) Antihistamines (diphenhydramine) at usual dosage of 10 to 50 mg over 5 minutes
6. Prevent further exposure to allergen
7. Monitor blood pressure because epinephrine may cause rapid increase

B. Treat allergic reaction without shock
1. Give oxygen via nasal prongs 3 to 6 L/min for pain
2. Administer medications
a) Epinephrine: subcutaneous (1:1,000 dilution) at usual dosage of 0.3 to 0.5 mg
b) Diphenhydramine (Benadryl): IM or IV at usual dosage of 10 to 50 mg

C. If reaction is the result of blood or medication infusion, stop administration and treat as described previously; follow hospital protocol for transfusion reaction; physician may decide to transfuse a different unit of blood along with antihistamines, epinephrine, and steroids, depending on need for blood

I. Secondary intervention
A. Provide comfort measures
1. Reassurance
2. Ice to local reaction
B. Inform family of patient progress

VALUATION

I. Patient outcomes/criteria
A. Vital signs within normal limits
B. Absence of respiratory distress
C. Improved mental status
D. Improvement of flushing, diaphoresis

II. Document initial assessment data, emergency department interventions, and patient's response to treatment

II. If previous patient outcomes are not reached, the emergency nurse should reevaluate the interventions and change the plan of care accordingly

DISPOSITION

I. Admission criteria
   A. Patient with anaphylactic shock
II. Discharge guidelines
   A. Give patient instructions
      1. Avoid contact with sensitizing agent, if known
      2. Return if reaction recurs
      3. Wear allergy alert bracelet when appropriate
   B. Give medications: patient may be sent home with antihistamine, e.g., diphenhydramine
   C. Arrange follow-up as indicated

CHAPTER 27

UNRESPONSIVE PATIENT

MPLICATIONS FOR ACTION

he unresponsive patient offers a challenge to emergency department person-el. Such patients require immediate attention with initial priorities directed ward airway management and hemodynamic stabilization. The patient is to-lly dependent on medical personnel. Assessment is then aimed at isolating e specific etiology. The following protocol outlines the initial priorities for re.

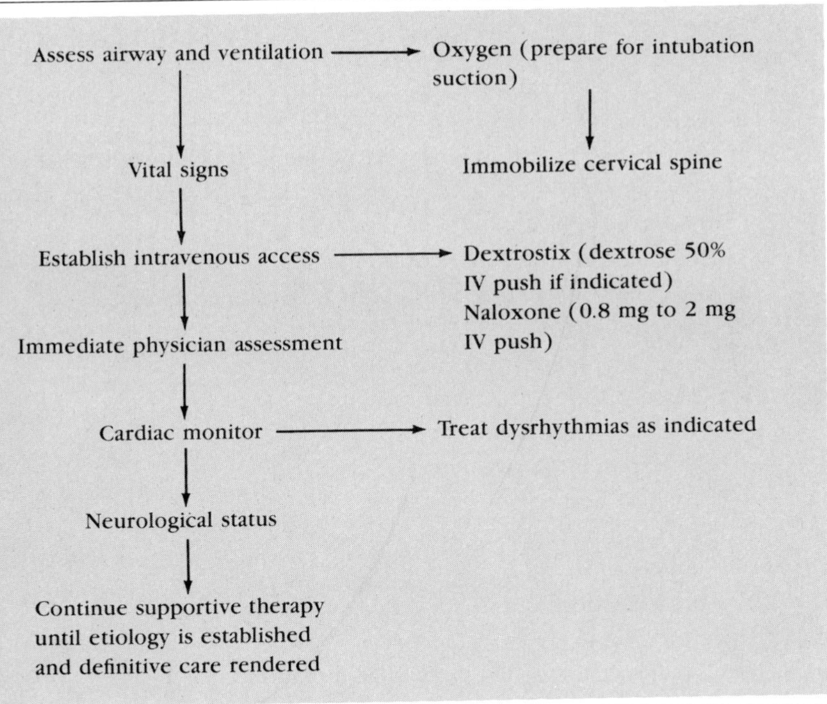

ASSESSMENT

I. Initial observation
   A. Level of consciousness
   B. Respiratory effort
   C. Skin color

II. Subjective assessment
   A. Information should be obtained from family, witnesses, and prehospit care providers
   B. History of episode
      1. How and where patient was found
      2. Time patient was last seen
      3. Environmental clues, such as medication bottles, alcohol, extrem cold or hot temperature, evidence of trauma

III. Objective assessment
   A. Patient must have clothes removed for adequate assessment
   B. Complete vital signs should be obtained, including rectal temperatur
   C. Respiratory status
      1. Patient arriving not intubated (refer to Chapter 22, Care Plan fo Respiratory Distress for indications when to intubate)
         a) Patency of airway
         b) Respiratory effort and rate, pattern, and quality
         c) Bilateral breath sounds
      2. Patient arriving intubated
         a) Bilateral breath sounds with assisted or spontaneous ventilation
         b) Position and security of endotracheal tube should be checked
   D. Cardiovascular status
      1. Skin color, temperature, and moisture
      2. Obvious wounds, bleeding, ecchymosis should be noted
   E. Neurological status
      1. Level of consciousness
      2. Response to noxious stimuli
         a) Reflex posturing
         b) Purposeful movement
      3. Pupil size and response to light
      4. Neurological assessment scale should be used, such as Glasgow Coma Scale
      5. Posturing: decerebrate, decorticate
   F. Odor of breath (alcoholic, ketotic)
   G. Neck stiffness, indicating meningeal irritation

H. Evidence of emesis or blood on clothes
I. Integrity of skull and scalp should be checked, noting any leakage of CSF from nose or ears

)SSIBLE NURSING DIAGNOSIS/ANALYSIS

I. Airway clearance, ineffective
II. Breathing pattern, ineffective
II. Cardiac output, alteration in: decreased
V. Fluid volume deficit, actual
V. Injury: potential for
I. Gas exchange, impaired
I. Tissue perfusion, alteration in: cerebral, cardiopulmonary

ANNING

Priorities for care
A. Airway management
B. Hemodynamic stabilization
C. Isolating cause of altered neurological status

Differential management

pe	Clinical Assessment	Management
ASCULAR TRAUMA		
ried Etiologies	Ruptured intracranial aneurysm, cerebral embolus or occlusion, ruptured cerebral vessel; asymmetry of body movements, receptive or expressive speech disturbances; patient may have had previous complaints of headache, dizziness, altered mental status, local neurological deficits, seizure activity, signs of increased intracranial pressure	Manage airway; hyperventilate to lower P_{CO_2} and thus cerebral blood volume; arrange for CT scan or angiography; administer diuretics if intracranial pressure is increased; hospital admission may be necessary
ypertensive ıcephalopathy	Malignant hypertension may cause loss of autoregulation of cerebral blood flow, edema, and increased intracranial pressure	Administer antihypertensive agents to allow controlled, not rapid, decrease in blood pressure (refer to Chapter 12, Care Plan for Headache for specific management)

Type	Clinical Assessment	Management
CEREBRAL TRAUMA		
Varied Etiologies	Epidural, subdural, subarachnoid or intracerebral hemorrhage resulting from head injury, concussion, cerebral edema; signs of increased intracranial pressure: decreased level of consciousness, pupillary changes, bradycardia, hypertension, altered respiratory patterns; hyperthermia	Hyperventilate and oxygenat administer medications to decrease intracranial pressure; diuretic or steroid (see Implementation section in this care plan for medications); perform CT scan, skull x-ray study; neurosurgical admission may be necessary
TOXIC TRAUMA		
Varied Etiologies	Acute poisoning: alcohol, carbon monoxide, barbiturate, tricyclic antidepressant, hypnotic agents, lead (encephalopathy), cyanide, opiates	(Refer to Care Plans for Chapter 2, Alcohol Intoxication; Chapter 20, Poisoning; and Chapter 33, Inhalation Injuries)
METABOLIC TRAUMA		
Hypoglycemia Hyperglycemia	Diabetic ketoacidosis and hyperosmolar nonketotic coma	(Refer to Chapter 6, Care Pla for Diabetic Emergencies); observe for alterations in blood glucose
Alcoholic Ketoacidosis	(Refer to Chapter 6, Care Plan for Diabetic Emergencies)	
Hyponatremia	Muscle twitches, seizures, motor weakness, lethargy, coma; cellular water intoxication	Administer hypertonic saline; control fluid and electrolytes, provide cardiac monitoring
Hypernatremia/ Hyperosmolarity	Signs of dehydration; mental status changes to coma	Treat underlying disorder; correct slowly by IV of dextrose 5%; rapid hydration can cause sudden osmotic gradient into cell, causing i to swell
Hepatic Encephalopathy	Enlarged liver and spleen; neurological progression of altered mental status, agitation, and coma; asterixis; seizures; jaundice	Determine ammonia levels; perform liver function tests administer lactulose 20-30 gm PO t.i.d. to diminish formation of ammonia

pe	Clinical Assessment	Management
enal Failure	Increased blood urea, nitrogen, and creatinine; weight loss; altered mental status; hypertension; acidosis; hyperkalemia	Perform dialysis
ypercapnea or ypoxemia	Results from hypoventilation	Provide ventilatory support; treat underlying disorder
NDOCRINE TRAUMA		
ypocalcemia	Muscle cramps, tetany, seizure activity, dysrhythmias	Administer intravenous calcium; patient may also have hypomagnesemia
ypercalcemia	Fatigue, gastrointestinal disorders, history of kidney stones, renal failure	Infuse with saline; parathyroid surgery may be necessary
ypothyroidism	Decreased metabolic activity, hypotension, bradycardia, hypothermia, inadequate ventilation, dysrhythmias	Provide respiratory support; obtain T_3, T_4, and BH levels; patient may receive IV steroids and levothyroxine
ypopituitarism	May result from head trauma or follow neurosurgery, diabetes insipidus (antidiuretic deficiency)	Diagnose with serum cortisol; treat with glucocorticoids
NFECTIOUS TRAUMA		
erebral Abscess	Fever, headache, visual changes, seizures	Administer antibiotics; perform CT scan
eningeal ncephalitis	Headache, nuchal rigidity, fever, irritability, photophobia	Assist with lumbar puncture, administer antibiotic therapy, perform hydration
epsis	Can cause unresponsiveness if patient becomes hypotensive; patient may have fever and chills; tachycardia	Initiate hydration; isolate source of infection with cultures of urine, blood, sputum; assist with lumbar puncture; administer antibiotic therapy
UMOR		
erebral Tumor resulting in erebral edema)	History of altered mental status, personality changes, visual disturbances, ataxia, seizures, headache, vomiting	Perform CT scan; administer steroids; arrange for neurosurgical care

Type	Clinical Assessment	Management
PSYCHOGENIC TRAUMA		
Catatonia or Conversion Reaction		Must rule out organic etiology for unresponsiveness; arrange psychiatric care
ENVIRONMENTAL TRAUMA		
Hypo- or Hyperthermia	(Refer to Care Plans for Chapter 15, Hypothermia and Chapter 14, Hyperthermia)	
NUTRITIONAL TRAUMA		
	Consider Wernicke's encephalopathy in poorly nourished alcoholic patient, caused by thiamine deficiency (thiamine facilitates glucose metabolism); ataxia, nystagmus, or ocular palsies may occur; mental status changes progressing to coma	Administer thiamine 100 mg intravenously, then 50-100 mg IV or IM every day until patient resumes normal diet; hydrate with dextrose and saline; also give magnesium 2 gm IM (50%)
SHOCK		
	All etiologies of shock result in insufficient delivery of oxygen and metabolites to and from the cell; often difficult to isolate etiology in unresponsive patient	Assess coma response to fluid challenge; solicit any available history
Hypovolemic	Traumatic hemorrhage; gastrointestinal bleeding; plasma loss (from burns); sequestering third space (ascites); extensive diuresis	Initiate hydration

pe	Clinical Assessment	Management
rdiogenic	May be accompanied by pulmonary edema	Institute vasopressor therapy: controlled vasodilator therapy may also be used to decrease afterload (refer to Chapter 17, Care Plan for Medical Cardiopulmonary Arrest)
aphylactic	Allergic reaction	Flushed skin and hives may provide clue (refer to Chapter 26, Care Plan for Systemic Allergic Reaction)
ptic	Circulating endotoxin results in vasodilatation	Obtain cultures; administer antibiotics; provide hydration
eurogenic or sogenic	Result of spinal cord disease or trauma	(Refer to Chapter 38, Care Plan for Spinal Injury)
ISCELLANEOUS		
ostictal or Status izures	(Refer to Chapter 23, Care Plan for Seizures)	

IPLEMENTATION

. Primary intervention

A. Manage airway
   1. If ventilations are adequate, administer 4 to 6 L/min of oxygen via nasal prongs or mask
   2. If ventilations are inadequate, oxygenate patient with ambu-bag and mask and prepare for intubation
   3. Obtain arterial blood gases; correct acidosis with bicarbonate

B. Establish intravenous access
   1. Normal saline if patient considered hypovolemic
   2. 5% dextrose in water if patient has normal vital signs or is hypertensive; will depend on etiology

C. Monitor cardiac activity
   1. Treat dysrhythmias as appropriate
   2. (Refer to Chapter 17, Care Plan for Medical Cardiopulmonary Arrest)
   3. Obtain 12-lead ECG and check for any irregularities

D. Use dextrostix or chemstick to estimate glucose (give dextrose 50% 25 gm IV push if low)

E. Administer naloxone 0.8 mg to 2 mg IV push to rule out narcotic ove dose
F. Perform laboratory studies
   1. Hematocrit
   2. Electrolytes
   3. Glucose
   4. BUN, creatine
   5. Blood and urine toxicology screens
   6. Consider thyroid levels, serum osmolarity
   7. Arterial blood gases for cardiorespiratory compromise or if acidosi is suspected
G. Immobilize cervical spine if trauma is suspected
H. Perform chest, skull, and cervical spine x-ray studies to rule out traum
I. Insert indwelling urinary catheter and nasogastric tube if patient re mains unresponsive after initial interventions
J. Individualize care as outlined in the differential management section a end of care plan (such as CT scan, consults)
K. Administer medications
   1. Mannitol: usual dosage 0.5 to 2 gm/kg IV bolus; then infusion 0.15 t 0.39 gm/kg q1 hour
   2. Furosemide: usual dosage 0.3 to 1 mg/kg IV bolus
   3. Dexamethasone: usual dosage 10 mg IV bolus initially, then 6 mg q6h or 100 mg IV bolus, then 20 mg q6h
   4. Anticonvulsant therapy (refer to Chapter 23, Care Plan for Seizures)

II. Secondary intervention
   A. Perform serial assessment of vital signs, neurological status, and dys rhythmias
   B. Position patient to maintain patent airway
   C. Position patients who are unresponsive but not intubated on their side to avoid aspiration if vomiting occurs
   D. Maintain warm environment
   E. Offer information and support to family

EVALUATION

I. Patient outcomes/criteria
   A. Vital signs within normal limits
   B. Control of dysrhythmias
   C. Correction of acid/base balance and hypoxemia
   D. Improved level or maintenance of level of consciousness
   E. Control of seizure activity

F. Correction of altered electrolytes

G. Arterial blood gases within normal limits

. Document initial assessment, emergency department interventions, and patient's response to treatment

. If previous patient outcomes are not reached, the emergency nurse should reevaluate the interventions and change the plan of care accordingly

ISPOSITION

Admission criteria

A. Continued abnormal neurological examination or altered mental status

B. Most illnesses, except those with rapid response to treatment such as hypoglycemia or alcohol or rapidly metabolized drug intoxication

Discharge guidelines

A. Provide patient teaching regarding cause of illness

B. Give appropriate counseling for drug abuse patient

C. Outline criteria for when to seek medical treatment

D. Determine follow-up arrangements if appropriate

CHAPTER 28

VAGINAL BLEEDING

IMPLICATIONS FOR ACTION

A patient who has vaginal bleeding should have vital signs taken before a con plete history is elicited. If the patient is found to be orthostatic or hypotensiv the priorities are to restore the fluid deficit with IV hydration, obtain appropr ate laboratory data, and secure physician assessment. A more detailed histor can be obtained while these measures are being initiated.

ASSESSMENT

I. Initial observation
   A. Skin color
   B. Body position indicative of pain
   C. Blood-saturated clothing
II. Subjective assessment
   A. Gynecological history
      1. Gravida, para, abortions; differentiate spontaneous from therapeuti abortions
      2. Date of last menstrual period; duration and amount of flow
      3. Pregnancy suspected or confirmed; if confirmed, expected date o confinement (EDC)
      4. If patient is postpartum: date of delivery, complications of preg nancy or delivery
      5. Trauma from intercourse, sexual assault, or abortive attempts
      6. Type of contraceptive used, if any
      7. History of dysmenorrhea, dysfunctional uterine bleeding, or dys pareunia

B. Current bleeding
   1. Onset and duration
   2. Length of time for pad or tampon saturation
   3. Presence of clots or tissue

C. Associated symptoms
   1. Abdominal pain or cramping: generalized or localized
   2. Nausea, vomiting, diarrhea, constipation
   3. Dysuria, pyuria, hematuria, or flank pain
   4. Fever or chills
   5. Referred pain

. Objective assessment
   A. Vital signs with orthostatics
   B. Amount of current bleeding
   C. Skin color, temperature, diaphoresis

SSIBLE NURSING DIAGNOSES/ANALYSIS

I. Anxiety
II. Cardiac output, alteration in: decreased
III. Comfort, alteration in: pain
IV. Fluid volume deficit, actual or potential
V. Grieving, anticipatory
VI. Knowledge deficit (as to why having vaginal bleeding)
/II. Rape trauma syndrome
III. Spiritual distress (distress of the human spirit)

LANNING

Priorities for care
   A. Fluid management
   B. Identifying etiology of bleeding

Differential management (NOTE: All patients who have vaginal bleeding require as a first priority stabilization of vital signs with fluid management; the treatment protocols outlined in the following differential are procedures specific to the etiology of the bleeding)

Cause	Clinical Assessment	Management
THREATENED ABORTION		
	Mild to acute cramping with variable amount of bleeding; internal cervical os remains closed; cause usually unknown	Discharge with instructions for bedrest until bleeding stops; r turn if tissue is passed or bleeding increases
SPONTANEOUS OR INEVITABLE ABORTION		
	Mild to acute cramping with variable amount of bleeding and clots; may have passed tissue; internal os open as demonstrated by passage of sterile ring forceps	Curettage
ECTOPIC PREGNANCY		
	Mild to acute abdominal pain often localized, with or without vaginal bleeding; usually late menstrual period; patient may have orthostatic vital signs or hypovolemic shock	Obtain pregnancy test and ultrasound; assist with culdocentes (refer to appendix A for procedure and equipment); laparotomy usually performed
PLACENTA PREVIA		
	Result of placental attachment in lower uterine segment near or covering os; bleeding during third trimester, often around 8 months; usually without pain or contractions	Check fetal heart tones; may require emergency cesarean sec tion
ABRUPTIO PLACENTAE		
	Separation of area of placenta from uterine wall, resulting in varying amount of bleeding and pain; partial separation is evidenced by external bleeding; occult hemorrhage can be severe	Check fetal heart tones; emergency cesarean section
DYSFUNCTIONAL UTERINE BLEEDING		
	Usually the result of hormonal disturbances or failure to ovulate; irregular periods, spotting	Rule out other causes for vaginal bleeding, e.g., tumor, progesterone or birth control pills; curettage may be necessary

use	Clinical Assessment	Management
STPARTUM BLEEDING		
	Result of retained placental parts or thrombi detaching from placental sites and preventing normal involution of uterus; suspect if increase in vaginal bleeding is within 6 weeks of delivery	Administer oxytocin or methylergonovine maleate (Methergine); curettage; rule out sepsis
AUMA		
	May occur during intercourse, sexual assault, or abortive attempt	Suture lacerations; check for sepsis or peritonitis (refer to Chapter 37, Care Plan for Sexual Assault)
TRAUTERINE DEVICE (IUD)		
	May cause heavier than normal periods with varying amount of bleeding during cycle	Remove IUD; if inflammatory disease is present, treat with antibiotics
RCINOMA OF UTERUS		
	Patient may have spotting or hemorrhage	Arrange gynecological consult for workup and treatment
ORMAL MENSES		
	Patient may come to emergency department because of cramping or heavier than usual flow	Provide patient education; administer analgesia
TERINE FIBROIDS		
	Patient may have bleeding, pain, enlarged uterus; pregnancy test is negative or postmenopause	Arrange gynecological consult; patient may need stabilization for hypovolemia and urgent surgery
ISCELLANEOUS BLOOD DYSCRASIAS; OVARIAN DISEASE		
	Rare occurrences; patient has pain, bleeding disorders	Arrange appropriate medical or gynecological follow-up

IMPLEMENTATION

I. Primary intervention
   A. Provide IV hydration with normal saline or lactated Ringer's; indicate for orthostatic vital signs, hypotension, passage of tissue, or profus bleeding (i.e., saturating tampon or pad in 1 hour or less)
   B. Obtain laboratory data
      1. Determine baseline hematocrit
      2. Type and ascertain Rh for inevitable and spontaneous abortions
      3. Type and crossmatch for 2 to 4 units of whole blood if hematocrit <30% or patient is admitted to operating room
      4. Perform complete blood count and sedimentation rate if patient febrile; blood cultures if sepsis is suspected
      5. If urine pregnancy test is needed, patient will require catheterizatio as presence of blood in urine will cause false positive readings
      6. Obtain serum pregnancy test and ultrasound as indicated in diffe ential management section
   C. Prepare patient for pelvic examination
      1. Patient should empty bladder and rectum before examination
      2. Patient should be completely undressed and privacy should be pro vided
      3. Assemble the following equipment
         a) Speculum
         b) Sterile ring forceps
         c) Jumbo and regular cotton-tipped applicators
         d) Culture media and slides
         e) Sterile and nonsterile gloves
         f) Lubricant
      4. Assist and chaperone physician and offer support to patient durin pelvic examination
   D. Special procedures
      1. Curettage in emergency department
         a) Indicated after spontaneous abortion to remove retained tissu from the uterus
         b) Procedure
            (1) Obtain vital signs before and after procedure
            (2) Place patient in lithotomy position
            (3) Remove tissue from uterine lining by means of a curette o suction (refer to appendix A for procedure and equipment

(4) Administer medications
(*a*) Sedative and adequate analgesics: usually diazepam 10 mg and meperidine 50 mg slow IV push
(*b*) Oxytocin (Pitocin) may be added to IV fluid to control bleeding; usual concentration is 30 units/1000 ml
(*c*) Methylergonovine maleate (Methergine) 0.2 mg IM at end of procedure; patient will be discharged with instructions to continue oral methylergonovine maleate
(*d*) Anti-Rh immunoglobulin (RhoGAM or MICrhoGAM if less than 12-week gestation) if patient is Rh negative
(5) Evaluate postprocedural mental status and bleeding

2. Assist with culdocentesis
a) Diagnostic aid for hemoperitoneum; indicated when ectopic pregnancy is suspected
b) Procedure
(1) Rectum should be emptied before procedure, if possible; patient may need enema
(2) Position patient in lithotomy position and elevate head of bed to encourage pelvic pooling
(3) Have available local anesthetic, spinal needle, and culdocentesis tray (refer to appendix A)
(4) Aspiration from cul-de-sac
(*a*) Positive tap produces nonclotting blood with a hematocrit >15%; venous or arterial blood should clot
(*b*) Negative tap, defined by clear serous fluid, does not rule out ectopic pregnancy (may be unruptured)
(*c*) "Dry tap" is nondiagnostic

Secondary intervention

A. Take serial vital signs and repeat hematocrit if bleeding continues
B. Change sanitary napkin frequently to assess amount of bleeding
C. Provide for patient's privacy
D. Be supportive of expressions of fear or grief and allow interaction with family member or friend
E. Obtain psychiatric social services or clergy support for patient as appropriate

EVALUATION

I. Patient outcomes/criteria
   A. Decrease in bleeding
   B. Resolution of orthostasis
   C. Relief of pain or discomfort
   D. Relief of anxiety, fear, grief
II. Document initial assessment, emergency department interventions, ar patient's response to treatment
III. If previous patient outcomes are not reached, the emergency nurse shou reevaluate the interventions and change the plan of care accordingly

DISPOSITION

I. Admission criteria
   A. Patient with ectopic pregnancy
   B. Patient with complicated abortion (i.e., profuse bleeding, infection) (in advanced stages of pregnancy
II. Discharge
   A. Educate patient regarding etiology of vaginal bleeding
   B. Provide discharge instructions for threatened abortion or postcurettag (refer to appendix E)
   C. Give medication instructions
   D. Arrange for follow-up care

PART TWO

TRAUMA CARE PLANS

CHAPTER 29

CHILD ABUSE: NONACCIDENTAL TRAUMA

MPLICATIONS FOR ACTION

he possibility of child abuse often elicits uncomfortable feelings among nergency department staff. The fear of "accusing" innocent parents is intenfied by the difficulty in establishing a clear picture of nonaccidental trauma. ne responsibility is dual: the health of the child and the parent (remembering at the child is defenseless).

It is helpful to view the investigative process as beneficial not only to the hild but to the family as a whole. Through counseling and social service suprt, the parents or guardians may develop appropriate coping mechanisms, hich will lead to a more healthy home environment.

It is an ethical as well as legal responsibility to report any suspected child use case for further investigation. Errors in judgment, except neglect in rerting the incident, are not liable.

SSESSMENT

I. Initial observation
   - A. Note whether child is well nourished, clean, and adequately and appropriately dressed for environment
   - B. Observe interactions of child, parent or guardian, and staff

I. Subjective assessment
   - A. Attitude of parent or guardian
     1. Over-concern or lack of concern
     2. Defensiveness or anger
     3. Criticism of emergency department's care of child
     4. Rapid desire to leave department before visit is completed (NOTE: When a child has fallen or been injured at home, parents often feel guilty or neglectful, resulting in angry feelings or behavior; a non-

accusatory approach when eliciting history may give the parents opening to express their fears and guilt feelings)

B. Mechanism of injury
   1. Evaluate if mechanism is consistent with injury incurred
   2. Be alert to injury inconsistent with age of child, delay in seeki treatment, history of similar injuries, emergency department vis by injured siblings

C. Although children are often protective of abusive parents, valuable formation may be elicited if the child is interviewed alone

III. Objective assessment
   A. Vital signs including temperature
   B. Level of consciousness
      1. Appropriate behavior for age
      2. Orientation: can child tell name, is there orientation to time a place; if infant, does child respond to emergency department s roundings?
      3. In the older child, note a flat affect or failure to cry appropriatel
   C. Assessment of child, including present injury (NOTE: Many of the f lowing injuries are diagnosed by the physician, but it is wise for t nurse to be aware that abuse is a possible etiology)
      1. Skin lesions
         a) Characteristic signs of abuse or neglect: multiple lesions in va ing stages of healing
         b) Presence of surface injuries
            (1) Bruises on unusual areas of body such as upper arms or le and across back
            (2) Evidence of hair pulling such as bald patches
         c) Marks in shapes suggestive of assault
            (1) Bruises in cluster pattern of fingertips
            (2) Looped cord or strap marks
            (3) Circumferential markings as made by ropes or restraints
            (4) Human bites (crescent shaped)
         d) Burn injuries
            (1) Origin of burns inconsistent with activity appropriate child's age (e.g., a 1-year-old is not going to leap into a ba tub), location and pattern of burn, degree of burn
            (2) Most common burns include cigarette burns (which lea oval scars) found on hands, feet, and buttocks and whi may be mistaken for impetigo; scalding or dunking may al have been used as a form of punishment

2. Facial injuries
   a) Eyes: blunt trauma
      (1) Periorbital ecchymosis
      (2) Subconjunctival hemorrhage or acute hyphema
      (3) Dislocated lens or detached retina
      (4) Retinal hemorrhage (indicative of central nervous system injury)
   b) Nose
      (1) Deviated septum
      (2) Bleeding
   c) Mouth
      (1) Loosened or missing teeth or evidence of jaw fracture because of blunt trauma
      (2) Bruises on lips or lacerations of lip or tongue as a result of forced feedings
      (3) Bruises on side of mouth or surface abrasions caused by forcible gagging to silence or punish
   d) Ear
      (1) Blunt trauma, such as bruised earlobe, caused by twisting; "cauliflower" ear caused by repeated blows; ruptured eardrum
      (2) Hematoma behind tympanic membrane or bruising around mastoid indicative of basilar skull fracture
3. Head and central nervous system injuries
   a) Subdural hematoma; may result from forceful shaking or whiplash-type injury from hard blow
   b) Unexplained coma or seizures may be caused by increased intracranial pressure from swelling or bleeding
4. Chest
   a) Rib fractures
      (1) Deformity of chest
      (2) Limited mobility or respiratory difficulty
   b) Associated injuries include pneumothorax, hemothorax
5. Abdominal injuries
   a) Most common cause of death
   b) Blunt trauma
      (1) Liver or splenic injury may cause internal bleeding
      (2) Bruised or ruptured viscera, with associated pain, signs of shock, and peritoneal signs

6. Long-bone fractures
   a) Extremity deformity
   b) X-ray studies may indicate previous fractures

POSSIBLE NURSING DIAGNOSES/ANALYSIS

I. Child
   A. Comfort, alteration in: pain
   B. Communication, impaired: verbal
   C. Nutrition, alteration in: less than body requirements
II. Parent
   A. Coping, ineffective: family and individual, potential for growth
   B. Parenting, alteration in: actual or potential
   C. Violence, potential for self-directed or directed at others
III. Both
   A. Anxiety
   B. Self-concept, disturbance in: parent, child, or both
   C. Social isolation

PLANNING

I. Priorities for care
   A. Treating life-threatening injuries
   B. Treating specific injuries
   C. Initiating report of suspected nonaccidental trauma
II. Differential management

Types of Abuse	Characteristics	Management
NEGLECT		
	Child may be unbathed, poorly nourished, inadequately dressed for weather, wearing old or torn clothing	Refer to family crisis center and/or admit for hospitalizati
PHYSICAL ABUSE		
	Obvious physical signs of abuse; conflicting stories about accident; injury inconsistent with history	(Refer to appropriate Care Plans for Injuries); refer to family c sis center

pes of ɒuse	Characteristics	Management
XUAL ABUSE		
	Usually no obvious signs; child most likely to be physically well cared for; child may exhibit evidence of oral/anal penetration, as well as genital contact	(Refer to Chapter 37, Care Plan for Sexual Assault, as appropriate); refer to family crisis center
IOTIONAL ABUSE		
	Failure on part of parents to provide emotional support necessary to develop a sound personality, such as failure to thrive; also seen when teachers set children up to fail in school	Refer to family crisis center for further workup

IPLEMENTATION

Primary intervention

A. (Refer to other care plans as indicated for specific injuries)

B. Child must be totally undressed for examination

C. When possible, identify abusive parent or person and protect child as necessary in the emergency department

Secondary intervention

A. Notify physician and local authorities if initial assessment arouses suspicion of nonaccidental trauma or neglect
   1. The nurse is required or authorized by state law to report suspected nonaccidental trauma; no liability is incurred for a report made in error based on suggestive examination; the nurse cannot leave this responsibility to the physician's judgment alone; if, in the nurse's judgment, nonaccidental trauma is suspected, the authorities should be notified
   2. Attitude of staff should not be accusatory but supportive and nonthreatening

B. Notify local social service agency (e.g., Family Crisis Service) to obtain assistance for child and parents
   1. Family should be informed of actions being taken
   2. Child may be placed under custody of police or Family Crisis Service pending investigation

EVALUATION

I. Patient outcomes/criteria
   A. Vital signs within normal limits
   B. Arrangements for follow-up have been made
II. Document initial assessment data, emergency department interventio and patient's response to treatment
III. If previous patient outcomes are not reached, the emergency nurse sho reevaluate the interventions and change the plan of care accordingly

DISPOSITION

I. Admission criteria
   A. Significant injury that warrants admission
   B. Admission may be a protective interim measure, less threatening th police hold, pending social services or judicial investigation
II. Discharge guidelines
   A. Give follow-up instructions for injury
   B. Provide resource facilities and phone numbers to patient and family
   C. Arrange for continued investigation through social service agency

CHAPTER 30

EAR, NOSE, AND THROAT INJURIES

IPLICATIONS FOR ACTION

ar, nose, and throat (ENT) trauma in this care plan includes injuries to those ructures as well as a discussion of foreign body insult. Often injuries of the ar, nose, or throat occur in conjunction with other injuries; the life-threaten- g injury must be stabilized first.

Additionally, foreign body problems are a common problem in emergency epartments. Foreign bodies have a potential to produce a spectrum of clinical onditions from no symptoms to death.

SSESSMENT

I. Initial observation
   A. Respiratory status
   B. Level of consciousness
   C. Any obvious injury
I. Subjective assessment
   A. History of event producing injury
      1. Mechanism and circumstances surrounding injury
         a) Speed in accidents
         b) Description of forces
      2. Location and quality of pain
      3. History of any associated loss of consciousness with injury or vertigo
      4. History of any partial or complete deafness, vertigo
      5. If foreign body, any attempts at removal
      6. If foreign body in airway, history of episode of violent coughing or salivation followed by asymptomatic interval possible

7. If foreign body, establish nature of (obtain duplicate if possible)
   a) Metal/plastic
   b) Sharp/dull
   c) Shape

B. Pertinent medical history
   1. Previous ENT trauma or disorders
   2. History of impaired hearing
   3. Other medical problems, history of vertigo
   4. Medications, allergies
   5. Tetanus status

C. Related injuries
   1. Concussion
   2. Skull fractures
   3. Cervical spine fractures

D. If pediatric patient or family cannot explain injury, consider possib child abuse

III. Objective assessment

A. Complete vital signs

B. Respiratory status
   1. Any loose material and developing edema should be noted; list carefully for noisy breathing
   2. Ability to speak and quality of vocalization

C. Neurological status
   1. Level of consciousness
   2. Observe nasal and ear drainage for presence of CSF leakage*
   3. Presence of mastoid or periorbital ecchymosis

D. Cardiovascular status
   1. Any obvious source of bleeding

E. Characteristics of wound
   1. Obvious arterial or venous bleeding
   2. Location and depth of wound
   3. Visible underlying structures
   4. Extent of wound contamination or foreign body presence
   5. Local inflammatory response or necrotic tissue

F. Auditory assessment: gross hearing check by using watch, tuning fo or snap of breaking applicator stick

G. Facial nerve function: if diminished or absent, injury to facial nerve middle ear is possible as result of foreign body or attempts to remov

---

*Notify physician immediately, if suspected.

POSSIBLE NURSING DIAGNOSES/ANALYSIS

I. Airway clearance, ineffective
II. Anxiety
III. Breathing pattern, ineffective
IV. Comfort, alteration in: pain
V. Skin integrity, impairment of: actual
VI. Knowledge deficit (related to injury)

PLANNING

I. Priorities for care
   A. Control and maintenance of airway, breathing, and circulation (ABCs)
   B. Control of bleeding
   C. Removal of foreign body
   D. Cleansing and repair of wounds
II. Differential management

Condition	Clinical Assessment	Management
EAR		
Foreign Body in Ear Canal	Pain on elevating ear; diminished or absent facial nerve function; foreign body visualized; patient may be dizzy (more common in pediatrics); may complain of buzzing when foreign body is insect	Avoid instilling or irrigating ear unless tympanic membrane is intact; never irrigate vegetable matter since it will swell; referral to consultant for formal operative removal may be necessary; drown insect in mineral oil
External Ear Trauma	Ecchymosis, localized bleeding, hematoma, fluctuant swelling, diminished hearing	For avulsions, saturate sponge with povidone-iodine and use to cover the area; wrap avulsed part in sponge saturated with normal saline and place in plastic bag and store over ice; any significant ear injury must be splinted in anatomical position using fluffed gauze for support and wrapping the head; NEVER use epinephrine anesthesia with ear lacerations since it can cause necrosis

Condition	Clinical Assessment	Management
Frostbite	Patient may complain of severe pain; observe for bleb formation	(Refer to Chapter 15, Care Pla[n] for Hypothermia)
NOSE		
Nasal Fractures	Usually follow blunt blow to face; decreased patency of nasal airways; edema; visual displacement of nose; epistaxis	Protect airway, rule out cervic[al] injury; control bleeding wit[h] direct nostril pressure; if po[s]sible, keep patient upright; use cold packs; refer to consultant; (refer to Chapter 9, Care Plan for Epistaxis as necessary)
Foreign Body in Nose	Most common site; history of placing object in nose; patient may have purulent, unilateral, malodorous nasal discharge	Assure patent airway; removal by physician is necessary
Epistaxis	(Refer to Chapter 9, Care Plan for Epistaxis)	
THROAT		
Foreign Body in Air Passages	Sudden respiratory distress while eating; obstruction at glottic area, cyanosis and death may ensue	Repeat Heimlich maneuver twice; manual removal by physician; prepare for cricothyrotomy (refer to appendi[x] A for procedure and equipment); prepare patient if sta[ble] for bronchoscopy; initiat[e] oxygen therapy as soon as possible
Tracheal or Laryngeal Injury; Pharyngeal Injury	(Refer to Chapter 34, Care Plan for Major Multiple Trauma)	
Caustic Substance Ingestion	(Refer to Chapter 20, Care Plan for Poisoning)	

PLEMENTATION

Primary intervention

A. Control and maintain airway
B. Maintain cervical spine immobilization as needed (refer to Chapter 34, Care Plan for Major Multiple Trauma)
C. Follow guidelines in differential management section of this care plan
D. Obtain intravenous access as necessary according to vital signs
E. Control any obvious hemorrhage (refer to Chapter 9, Care Plan for Epistaxis for nasal bleeding considerations)
F. Cleanse wound (refer to Chapter, 41, Care Plan for Wound Management)
G. Prepare patient for x-ray studies as ordered by physician

Secondary intervention

A. Reassure patient about temporary disfigurement
B. Monitor vital signs, neurological status, and respiratory status
C. Administer medications as indicated
   1. Analgesics
   2. Tetanus prophylaxis (refer to Chapter 41, Care Plan for Wound Management for tetanus schedule)
   3. Antibiotics as determined by physician
D. Treat associated problems and injuries as indicated

ALUATION

. Patient outcomes/criteria
   A. Improved respiratory status
   B. Bleeding controlled
   C. Relief of anxiety
   D. Relief of pain

. Document initial assessment data, emergency department interventions, and the patient's response to treatment

. If previous patient outcomes are not reached, the emergency nurse should reevaluate the interventions and change the plan of care accordingly

SPOSITION

. Admission criteria
   A. Patients with recurrent or persistent hemorrhage
   B. Patients requiring blood transfusions

II. Discharge guidelines
   A. Give patient instructions
      1. Cold packs to all nasal fractures
      2. Cautions same as for epistaxis patients
      3. Wound care same as for facial trauma patient
         a) Keep wounds clean and dry
         b) Return to emergency department if there is redness, swelli draining pus, chills, fever
         c) Keep head elevated to promote drainage, reduce swelling, a decrease pain
   B. Explain follow-up
      1. When to return for follow-up
      2. Final therapeutic results often will taken 6 months for resolutior

CHAPTER 31

EYE INJURIES

IMPLICATIONS FOR ACTION

Injuries to the eye are a common problem seen in all emergency departments. As in any case of facial trauma, the emergency nurse's attention must be directed to those injuries that are life threatening.

If the eye-injured patient complains of suddenly seeing floaters—moving spots, lightning flashes, or sparks—this may indicate a retinal detachment. Keep patient's head immobilized, patch both eyes, and have physician see patient immediately. Caustic burns to eye also require immediate interventions:

1. Checking and removing contact lens
2. Copious irrigation of burned eye for at least 10 minutes before further assessment
3. Patient may need local and parenteral eye relief

ASSESSMENT

I. Initial observation
   A. Appearance of eye: laceration, foreign body, burn, redness, or tearing
   B. Other injuries to face
   C. Level of consciousness
II. Subjective assessment
   A. History of injury: including how and when it happened
   B. Alterations in vision: blurring, diplopia, photophobia, floating spots, flashes of light, blindness, cloudy or smoky vision
   C. Pain associated with injury
   D. Pertinent medical history
      1. Previous eye disorders or injuries; use of contact lenses, glasses, or prosthesis
      2. Other medical problems such as diabetes, hypertension
      3. Allergies, medications, and immunization status

III. Objective assessment
   A. Complete vital signs
   B. Physical assessment
      1. Foreign body, burn, ulcer, injected sclera, subconjunctival hemorrhage
      2. Blood or pus in anterior chamber, fullness of anterior chamber
      3. Pupil equality, shape, reactivity
      4. Obviously soft or malshaped globe
      5. Bloody or clear fluid leakage, presence of tearing
      6. Ocular mobility
   C. Visual acuity
      1. Ability to discern light and shapes
      2. Snellen chart: test each eye individually
   D. Evidence of other associated injuries
      1. Ecchymosis
      2. Edema
      3. Laceration of eyelid or surrounding structures
      4. Crepitus or deformity of bony orbit
      5. Burns

POSSIBLE NURSING DIAGNOSES/ANALYSIS

I. Anxiety
II. Comfort, alteration in: pain
III. Coping, ineffective individual
IV. Fear
V. Mobility, impaired physical
VI. Sensory-perceptual alteration: visual
VII. Knowledge deficit (related to injury)

PLANNING

I. Priorities for care
   A. Prevention of further damage
   B. Pain control
   C. Relief of anxiety
II. Differential management

e	Clinical Assessment	Management
ACTURES		
bital wout ctures	Diplopia, sunken eyeball; inability to elevate eye; decreased sensation on the affected cheek; pain on the affected side when looking up; subconjunctival hemorrhage; restricted extraocular movements in the affected eye; periorbital edema	Obtain visual acuity; if eye is not ruptured or does not have hyphema, apply ice pack; may need surgical intervention 7 to 10 days after hospital admission to release entrapped orbital muscles
UNT TRAUMA		
phema	Pain, report of seeing reddish tint	Test visual acuity, then place patient on stretcher in semi-Fowler's position, if able; patch both eyes; arrange ophthalmology consult
NETRATING INJURY		
	Pain, bleeding, profuse lacrimation, decreased visual acuity; visible corneal or scleral wound	DO NOT remove any impaled objects; DO NOT manipulate eyeball; place metal shield over eye; if patient is a child, may need to apply hand restraints; obtain intravenous access; administer systemic antibiotics, tetanus; arrange ophthalmology consult and hospitalization
HEMICAL BURNS OF THE EYE		
	Eye pain; absence of pain usually indicates severe damage; inability to keep eye open; impaired vision	Perform immediate copious irrigation until conjunctival pH reaches 7; test visual acuity; arrange ophthalmology consult
ORNEAL FOREIGN BODIES, ABRASIONS, AND LACERATIONS		
	Patient will complain of something in eye and have eyelid spasm, squinting, blinking, profuse lacrimation, diminished pupil size, photophobia, decreased visual acuity	Check visual acuity; place patient in darkened room; check and remove contact lens; remove foreign body by flushing with normal saline; arrange ophthalmology consult
ADIATION BURNS (from sun lamps, welding arcs, etc.)		
	Delayed symptoms of pain, excessive lacrimation	Patch and administer analgesics to relieve pain

IMPLEMENTATION

I. Primary intervention
   A. Check patient's visual acuity first, except in the case of chemical burn
      1. Check eyes separately with Snellen chart
      2. Physician may need to anesthetize eye
   B. Irrigate eye(s) for chemical burns
      1. Place patient supine and turn head to affected side
      2. Do not stream fluid directly onto pupil
      3. Encourage intermittent blinking to distribute fluid
   C. Place patient at rest supine or in semi-Fowler's position
   D. Do not remove foreign bodies or apply pressure to the globe or allo patient to blow nose
   E. Apply sterile dressing for bleeding; patch eyes as ordered; do not wip away clots
   F. Remove contact lenses in the unconscious patient
   G. Place side rails up; many patients have distorted depth perception
   H. Follow guidelines in differential management section

II. Secondary intervention
   A. Physician usually examines and treats patient
      1. Fluorescein stain and Wood's lamp evaluation for corneal abrasion o laceration
      2. Tonometry for suspected increased or decreased ocular pressure
      3. Instillation of drops: anesthetics, mydriatics, cycloplegics, or ant biotics
      4. Evaluation of integrity of internal structures
   B. Obtain x-ray studies for fractures or metallic foreign bodies
   C. Obtain coagulation studies for hyphema
   D. Administer parenteral analgesia or sedation as ordered
   E. Provide reassurance
   F. Culture purulent drainage

'ALUATION

. Patient outcomes/criteria
  A. Improvement in vision or no further deterioration
  B. Relief of anxiety
  C. Relief of pain
. Document initial assessment data, emergency department interventions, and patient's response to treatment
. If previous patient outcomes are not reached, the emergency nurse should reevaluate the interventions and change the plan of care accordingly

'SPOSITION

Admission criteria
A. Hyphema
B. Any penetrating injuries
C. Orbital fractures with entrapment
D. Traumatic blindness
E. Retinal detachment

Discharge guidelines
A. Provide instructions
  1. Explain damage to eye
  2. Explain physician instruction regarding activity and follow-up
  3. Warn patient of loss of depth perception with eye patch
  4. Discuss any other physician instructions
B. Arrange follow-up
  1. Appointment with ophthalmologist as indicated

CHAPTER 32

FACIAL INJURIES

IMPLICATIONS FOR ACTION

Facial trauma in this care plan includes injuries to the soft tissues of the fac and to facial bone structure. Dental trauma will also be discussed.

The emergency care rendered to patients with facial injuries can affect th final therapeutic result a patient achieves. Since facial trauma often occurs i conjunction with other injuries, the life-threatening injuries must be stabilize first.

ASSESSMENT

I. Initial observation
   A. Respiratory status
   B. Level of consciousness
   C. Any obvious injuries
II. Subjective assessment
   A. History of event producing injury
      1. Mechanism and circumstances surrounding injury (incidents unde police investigation can cause decreased patient cooperation)
         a) Velocities of accident vehicles
         b) Description of forces involved, such as hand, tire iron, etc.
   B. Location of pain, quality of pain
   C. Associated symptoms
      1. History of any associated loss of consciousness with injury
      2. History of any partial or complete deafness or visual loss
      3. Decreased sensation changes
   D. Pertinent medical history
      1. Previous facial trauma
      2. Medications, allergies
      3. Tetanus status
      4. History of keloid formation

E. Predisposing risk factors: young adult males; persons involved in high speed accidents, fast-moving machinery work, with high velocity missiles; patients with seizure disorders; patients involved in motorcycle, bicycle, or snowmobile accidents
F. Related injuries
   1. Concussion
   2. Skull fracture
   3. Cervical spine fracture
   4. Other fractures, especially long bones
G. If pediatric patient or patient's family cannot explain how injury occurred or the mechanism involved, consider child abuse

I. Objective assessment
   A. Complete vital signs
   B. Respiratory status: look for loose material and developing edema; if patient is breathing adequately, listen carefully for noisy breathing—can herald obstruction
   C. Cardiovascular status
      1. Any obvious source of bleeding should be noted
   D. Neurological status
      1. Level of consciousness
      2. Check pupil size and reactivity
      3. Check nasal and ear drainage for presence of CSF; use a dipstick and check the glucose—a positive result is indicative of CSF leakage (NOTIFY PHYSICIAN IMMEDIATELY)
      4. Presence of mastoid or periorbital ecchymosis
      5. Sensation
      6. Motion: ability of patient to raise eyebrows, squeeze eyes, wrinkle nose
   E. Check facial symmetry: palpate for tenderness, bony defects, crepitus, false motion
   F. Characteristics of wound
      1. Obvious arterial or venous bleeding
      2. Location and depth of wound
      3. Edema, swelling
      4. Visible underlying structures
      5. Extent of wound contamination or foreign body presence
      6. Local inflammatory response or necrotic tissue
   G. Analyze injury: is apparent trauma consistent with mechanism of injury? Assume worst injury until proven otherwise

POSSIBLE NURSING DIAGNOSES/ANALYSIS

I. Airway clearance, ineffective
II. Anxiety
III. Breathing pattern, ineffective
IV. Comfort, alteration in: pain
V. Oral mucous membranes, alteration in
VI. Skin integrity, impairment of: actual
VII. Sensory-perceptual alteration: visual, gustatory, olfactory

PLANNING

I. Priorities for care
  A. Control and maintenance of airway, breathing, and circulation (ABCs)
  B. Control of bleeding
  C. Cleansing and repairing wounds
II. Differential management

Type	Clinical Assessment	Management
FACIAL FRACTURES		
Mandibular Fractures	Second most common type after nasal; patient complains of pain and teeth not fitting together; trismus	Maintain airway; obtain intravenous access; surgical intervention may be necessary
Temporomandibular Joint Dislocation	Jaw is displaced forward and superiorly; patient cannot close/open mouth and usually is in pain	Manual relocation by physician or oral surgeon in emergency department
Zygomatic Fractures	Edema to inferior rectus muscle of eye causing lack of consensual gaze; asymmetry of face, persistent trismus, chronic contraction of chewing muscles	Patient usually discharged from emergency department and hospitalized if necessary later for open reduction
Orbital Blowout Fracture	(Refer to Chapter 31, Care Plan for Eye Injuries)	
Nasal Fracture	(Refer to Chapter 30, Care Plan for Ear, Nose, and Throat Injuries)	

pe	Clinical Assessment	Management
nus Fractures		
Frontal	Occurs with severe blows to forehead	Place patient in head-up position; refer to consultant for repair
Ethmoid	Blow to bridge of nose—cerebrospinal fluid (CSF) leak masked by epistaxis; traumatic epistaxis usually short lived, consider CSF leak if bleeding is persistent and liquid with few clots	Patient usually admitted to hospital in head elevated position; refer to consultant for repair
axillary ractures	Usually caused by motor vehicle crash or blunt trauma; massive force needed to produce fracture Classified as: 1. LeFort I: Fracture at nasal fossa, patient cannot close mouth 2. LeFort II: Fracture of maxilla, nasal bones, and medial orbits; nose moves with upper dental arch; concealed bleeding may cause gastric distention and nausea 3. LeFort III: Fracture of maxilla, zygoma, nasal bones, and ethmoid creating cranial dysfunction; patients have elongated face, extensive bleeding, tenuous airway; CSF leak	Active airway management may be necessary; head elevated if cervical spine "cleared"; apply cold packs; obtain intravenous access; antibiotics may be ordered; surgical internal fixation may be necessary
NJURIES TO FACIAL NERVE AND PAROTID SALIVARY GLAND		
	Injuries to cheek between tragus of ear and midcheek; must be suspected of injuring parotid salivary gland, facial nerve, or parotid duct; patient will lose motor function and sensation below level of injury	Motor examination needed by physician before use of any anesthetic; usually referred to consultant

Type	Clinical Assessment	Management
BURNS		
	(Refer to Care Plans for Chapter 41, Wound Management and Chapter 31, Eye Injuries for burns to eye)	
LACERATIONS		
	(Refer to Care Plans for Chapter 41, Wound Management and Chapter 31, Eye Injuries for burns to eye)	
BITES		
	(Refer to Chapter 41, Care Plan for Wound Management)	
DENTAL FRACTURES AND AVULSIONS		
	Patient will complain of pain, missing tooth; obvious chipped or avulsed teeth	Rule out aspiration of teeth; refer to dentist

IMPLEMENTATION

I. Primary intervention
   A. Control and maintain airway; if patient is apneic or in respiratory distress and endotracheal intubation is contraindicated, prepare for cricothyrotomy (refer to Chapter 34, Care Plan for Major Multiple Trauma and appendix A for procedure and equipment)
   B. Maintain cervical spine immobilization until x-ray studies are "cleared" (refer to Chapter 34, Care Plan for Major Multiple Trauma); cervical spine injury must be ruled out in the unconscious or inebriated patient and considered in all others
   C. Follow guidelines in differential management section
   D. Obtain intravenous access according to vital signs
   E. Control any obvious hemorrhage with pressure dressing (avoid blind use of instrument clamps); elevate head of bed 45 degrees IF cervical spine is stable; if patient is in shock, look for other sources of bleeding

F. Check patient's visual acuity as appropriate

G. Cleanse wounds (refer to Chapter 41, Care Plan for Wound Management)

1. Special considerations in facial trauma
   - *a*) Irrigate copiously to preserve tissue viability
   - *b*) Put any avulsed parts such as ears, nose, teeth in normal saline–soaked sponges placed in plastic bags and stored over ice
   - *c*) DO NOT use hydrogen peroxide to scrub wound
   - *d*) NEVER shave eyebrows
   - *e*) Mark vermillion border of lips before irrigation and anesthetizing

H. Prepare patient for x-ray studies as ordered by physician

Secondary intervention

A. Provide psychological support because of the nature of injury and because the face is such a prime focus for others

B. Monitor vital signs, neurological status, and respiratory status

C. Administer medications as indicated

1. Analgesics
2. Tetanus prophylaxis
3. Antibiotics as determined by physician

D. Treat associated problems and injuries as indicated

VALUATION

I. Patient outcomes/criteria

A. Improved respiratory status

B. Bleeding controlled

C. Relief of anxiety

D. Relief of pain

I. Document initial assessment data, emergency department intervention, and the patient's response to treatment

I. If previous patient outcomes are not reached, the emergency nurse should reevaluate the interventions and change the plan of care accordingly

ISPOSITION

. Admission criteria

A. All those patients with injuries to

1. Parotid duct glands
2. Facial nerves
3. Moderate soft tissue loss
4. Extensive lacerations requiring debridement and accurate closure
5. Mandibular and maxillary fractures
6. LeFort fractures

II. Discharge guidelines
   A. Instructions to patient
      1. Keep wounds clean, dry, soft
      2. Return or call emergency department if there is redness, swelling, draining pus, chills, fever
      3. For mouth injuries, rinse oral cavity with half strength hydrogen peroxide t.i.d.
      4. Keep head elevated to promote drainage, reduce swelling, and decrease pain
   B. Follow-up instructions
      1. Advise patient when to return for suture removal
      2. Patients should be told that final result of treatment cannot be evaluated until 6 months following injury

HAPTER 33

INHALATION INJURIES

·LICATIONS FOR ACTION

alation injuries occur in a variety of settings—home accidents, fires, indus-
l chemical spills or explosions—and may range in severity from temporary
:omfort to life-threatening emergencies. Whatever the cause or the severity
he injury, the immediate concern is to ensure a patent airway and adequate
·genation.

·ESSMENT

Initial observation

A. Skin color

B. Respiratory effort

C. Level of consciousness

D. Presence of burns on face, head, neck, or chest

Subjective assessment

A. Mechanism of injury

B. Associated signs and symptoms

   1. Nausea/vomiting
   2. Dizziness
   3. Chest pain
   4. Headache
   5. Vision changes

C. Past medical history

   1. Existing lung disease
   2. Cigarette smoking
   3. Medications and allergies

D. Indications of possible child abuse

E. History of self-inflicted inhalation

Objective assessment

A. Complete vital signs

B. Level of consciousness; may be abnormal because of hypoxia

C. Respiratory effort
   1. Skin color
   2. Respiratory rate
   3. Use of accessory muscles
   4. Breath sounds
      a) Rales
      b) Wheezes
   5. Cough; note color of sputum

D. Refer to Chapter 39, Care Plan for Burns for other assessment data, appropriate

POTENTIAL NURSING DIAGNOSES/ANALYSIS

I. Airway clearance, ineffective
II. Anxiety
III. Breathing pattern, ineffective
IV. Fear
V. Gas exchange, impaired
VI. Knowledge deficit (of potential toxic fumes)

PLANNING

I. Priorities for care
   A. Adequate airway; patient may need intubation or cricothyrotomy
   B. Oxygenation
   C. Treatment of associated systemic problems (refer to Chapter 39, Ca Plan for Burns)
II. Differential management

Type	Clinical Assessment	Management
BURN INJURIES		
Thermal Injury (rare unless occurred with hot steam or explosive gas)	Respiratory distress, possible stridor; wheezing, facial burns	Administer humidified oxyge 100% by mask; patient ma need intubation and mechanical ventilation; obtain intravenous access, monito arterial blood gases, possib carboxyhemoglobin level; obtain chest x-ray study; administer nebulized racemic epinephrine to co trol local edema every 2-4 hours and bronchodilators

pe	Clinical Assessment	Management
noke ıhalation		
Carbon monoxide (CO) poisoning	(Refer to assessment below)	Initial management is the same for all degrees of poisoning; administer 100% oxygen by humidified nonrebreathing mask, monitor carboxyhemoglobin level
CO level <10%	Headache/irritability	(Initial treatment as above)
CO level 10-20%	Nausea and vomiting; decreased dexterity	(Initial treatment as above); in addition, monitor arterial blood gases; provide intravenous access and cardiac monitoring
CO level 20-30%	Confusion, lethargy; patient may have ST segment depression	(Initial treatment as above); with high carboxyhemoglobin level and pH <7.4, use hyperbaric oxygen; monitor carboxyhemoglobin levels with 0.5-10 while patient is on 100% oxygen
CO level >40%	Loss of consciousness; seizures	Patient may need intubation; administer diazepam, phenytoin
Smoke poisoning (chemical toxicants)	Cough; wheezing; air hunger; damaged mucosa sloughs and leads to tracheobronchitis, acute respiratory disease, and bacterial pneumonia	Administer 100% oxygen by mask; obtain intravenous access, cardiac monitoring, intubation if posioning is severe; administer bronchodilators, pulmonary toilet; monitor arterial blood gases; obtain chest x-ray study
OXIOUS GASES AND FUMES		
hlorine, mmonia, and ulfur Dioxide	These three gases are all very irritating to eyes/nose and therefore do not cause significant damage unless inhaled in a closed environment; manifestations include coughing and wheezing	Maintain patent airway; administer 100% oxygen by mask

Type	Clinical Assessment	Management
Phosgene	Nausea, dizziness, cough; chest pain, wheezing; shortness of breath; hemoptysis	Maintain patent airway; administer humidified oxygen 100% by mask
Nitrogen Oxides	Cough, shortness of breath, bronchitis may lead to chronic obstructive pulmonary disease; both of these gases are odorless and are likely to cause tissue damage	Administer bronchodilators, possibly steroids with nitrogen oxides; monitor chest x-ray study and arterial blood gases; perform spirometry for 24 hours
Cyanide (very uncommon but extremely lethal)	Headache, vertigo, anxiety, agitation, arrhythmias (as a result of hypoxia), tachypnea, apnea, shortness of breath, respiratory paralysis, coma, seizures; high anion gap with severe metabolic acidosis; flushed appearance, possibly the odor of almonds on breath	Administer 100% oxygen; perform cardiac monitoring; obtain intravenous access; employ Lilly antidote kit (refer to Chapter 20, Care Plan for Poisoning); correct acidosis; monitor arterial blood gases and venous gases, serum lactate, serum pyrovate, cyanide level, and thiocyanate level
PESTICIDES		
Organophosphates and Carbamates	(Dealt with together because of similar clinical manifestations and management); blurred vision, miosis, cough, chest tightness, dyspnea, increased secretions; bradycardia, hypotension; nausea, vomiting, diarrhea, increased sweating, salivation, lacrimation, bladder/bowel incontinence, headache, weakness, atoxia, irritability, progressing to coma, seizures; CNS effects more common with organophosphates	Provide supportive treatment of clinical manifestations (refer to Chapter 20, Care Plan for Poisoning); maintain airway and adequate oxygenation with 100% oxygen; provide cardiac monitoring, intravenous access, indwelling urinary catheter; monitor RBC cholinesterase level; administer medications: atropine, pralidoxime chloride, diazepam, and phenytoin

IPLEMENTATION

Primary intervention

A. Respiratory
   1. Maintain airway; patient may need intubation (cricothyrotomy usually not necessary)
   2. Oxygenate: 100% humidified oxygen by mask or mechanical ventilation; patient may need hyperbaric oxygen with high carbon monoxide levels

B. Monitor cardiac activity

C. Provide intravenous access; in patients with major burns refer to Chapter 39, Care Plan for Burns; otherwise provide peripheral line using dextrose 5% at a keep-open rate

D. Administer medications
   1. Oxygen
   2. Bronchodilators
      a) Metaproterenol sulfate (Alupent): 0.3 ml of 0.5 or 0.6% solution by nebulizer
      b) Aminophylline: 5.6 mg/kg IV as loading dose followed by 0.9 mg/kg/hr maintenance drip
   3. Anticonvulsants
      a) Diazepam
         (1) Adult: up to 10 mg IV push slowly
         (2) Pediatric: 0.1 to 0.3 mg/kg IV push slowly
      b) Phenytoin: 15 mg/kg IV push at rate of 0.5 mg/kg/min
   4. Anticholinergics/cholinesterase reactivators (used with pesticide inhalation)
      a) Atropine
         (1) Adult: 2 to 4 mg IV push q5 to 10 min until atropinization* occurs
         (2) Pediatric: 0.05 mg/kg IV push q5 to 10 min until atropinization occurs
      b) Pralidoxime chloride (Protopam)
         (1) Adult: 500 mg to 2 gm IV push at rate of 500 mg/min for 8 hours × 3 doses
         (2) Pediatric: 10 to 50 mg/kg IV push slow (less than 50 mg/min) for 8 hours × 3 doses

---

*Atropinization—drying of secretions, bowel/bladder ileus.

5. Lilly Cyanide Antidote Kit
   a) Amyl nitrite inhalant for 15 seconds, then rest 15 seconds (rest to prevent hypoxia)
   b) Sodium nitrite
      (1) Adult: 300 mg IV push at rate of 2.5 to 5 ml/min
      (2) Pediatric: 0.2 ml/kg, not to exceed 10 ml
   c) Sodium thiosulfate
      (1) Adult: 12.5 gm or 500 ml IV of a 25% solution
      (2) Pediatric: 7 gm/square meter of body surface area, not exceed 12.5 gm
   d) If signs and symptoms of poisoning reappear, repeat same proc dure using half the dosage
   e) Consider laboratory data as outlined in differential manageme section

II. Secondary intervention
   A. Monitor serial vital signs
   B. Perform pulmonary toilet
   C. Provide explanations to patient and family

EVALUATION

I. Patient outcomes/criteria
   A. Restoration of normal or adequate respiratory function as indicated b normal ABG values and respiratory parameters
   B. Absence of systemic poisoning effects
   C. Vital signs within normal limits
   D. Improved mental status

II. Document initial assessment data, emergency department intervention and patient's response to treatment

III. If previous patient outcomes are not reached, the emergency nurse shoul reevaluate the interventions and change the plan of care accordingly

DISPOSITION

I. Admission criteria
   A. Intensive care unit (ICU) admission for patients with artificial airway those requiring mechanical ventilation, cardiac monitoring, or clos observation
   B. Patients with airway tissue damage
   C. Patients requiring oxygen therapy

D. Most patients with inhalation injuries who will require monitoring for 24-48 hours for serial chest x-ray studies, ABGs, spirometry measurements, and pulmonary toilet treatment

. Discharge guidelines

A. Make follow-up arrangements
B. Provide medication instructions
C. Instruct patients in the safe use of chemicals if appropriate
D. Consult area poison center; provide patient with appropriate resource information if necessary

CHAPTER 34

MAJOR MULTIPLE TRAUMA

IMPLICATIONS FOR ACTION

Systems covered in this care plan are head trauma, spinal and neck traun chest trauma, abdominal trauma, abdominal trauma in the pregnant patie and major orthopedic trauma.

Knowledge, anticipation, assessment, and appropriate attention to prio ties are the keys to smooth, efficient resuscitations. The team approach trauma care involves a designated leader from both medical and nursing st and defined roles for all team members. This allows for numerous interve tions to be carried out simultaneously when the patient arrives.

A detailed differential management section is found at the end of the ca plan. The protocol on the opposite page outlines priorities for care of a patie with major trauma.

ASSESSMENT

I. Initial observation
   A. Respiratory status
   B. Level of consciousness
   C. Obvious injuries
   D. Paramedic interventions such as intubation, intravenous access, imm bilization of spine or extremities
II. Subjective assessment
   A. Report of incident from patient, paramedics, or witnesses
      1. Mechanism of injury
         a) Blunt
            (1) Auto accident
               (*a*) Driver or passenger
               (*b*) Use of seatbelt
               (*c*) Speed and mechanism of collision

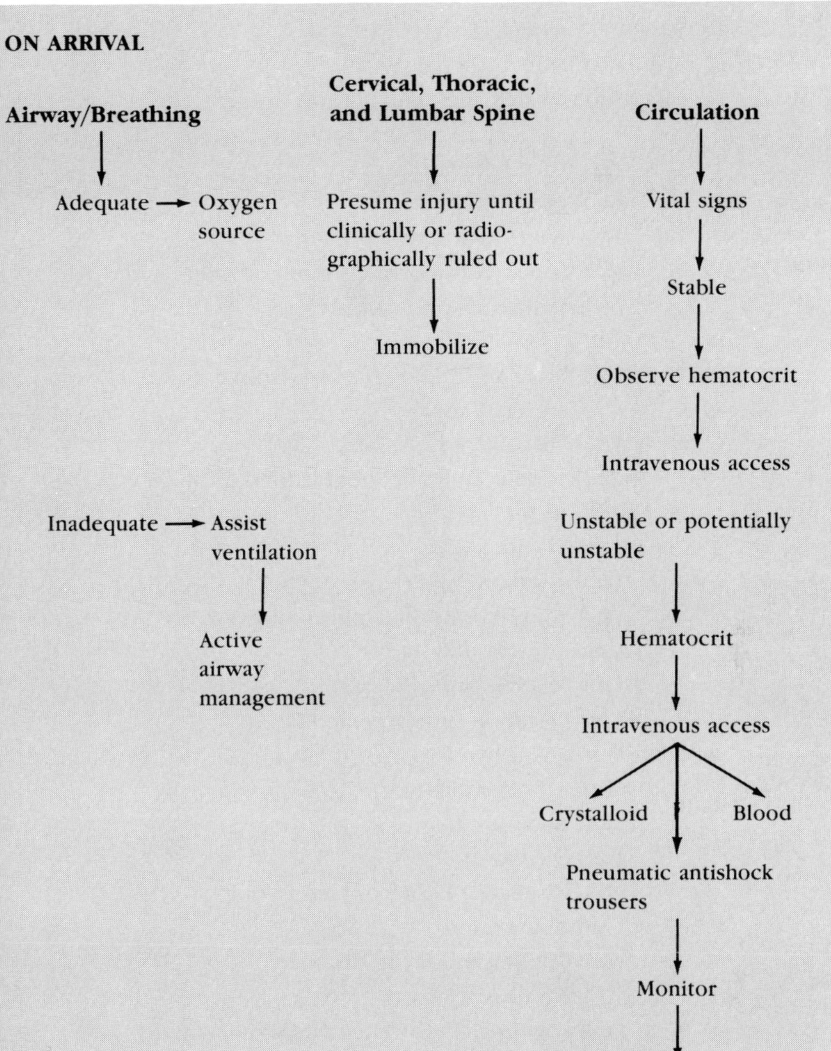
ON ARRIVAL
Airway/Breathing
Adequate → Oxygen source
Inadequate → Assist ventilation
Active airway management
Cervical, Thoracic, and Lumbar Spine
Presume injury until clinically or radiographically ruled out
Immobilize
Circulation
Vital signs
Stable
Observe hematocrit
Intravenous access
Unstable or potentially unstable
Hematocrit
Intravenous access
Crystalloid
Blood
Pneumatic antishock trousers
Monitor
Procedures to isolate the source of bleeding

(*d*) Damage to vehicle, especially windshield, steeri
wheel, dashboard
(*e*) Difficult extrication
(2) Motorcycle accident
(*a*) Speed and mechanism of collision
(*b*) Distance victim thrown
(*c*) Use of helmet
(3) Auto and/or pedestrian/cyclist
(*a*) Speed and mechanism of collision
(*b*) Distance victim thrown
(4) Fall
(*a*) Mechanism: down stairs, from a building, from a mo
ing vehicle
(*b*) Distance
(*c*) Type of object patient landed on such as cement, gra
water
(5) Assault
(*a*) Type of object used
(*b*) Number and location of blows
(6) Crush injury
(*a*) Mechanism of injury
(*b*) Duration of entrapment
b) Penetrating
(1) Type of object used
(2) Stab wound
(*a*) Direction
(*b*) Estimated depth of penetration
(3) Gunshot wound
(*a*) Caliber and firing distance
(*b*) Number of shots fired
(*c*) Location of entrance and exit wounds
(*d*) Presence of powder burns on skin or clothing
2. Loss of consciousness
3. Patient's memory of incident
B. Location and description of pain
C. Allergies, tetanus status, and medications
D. Pertinent medical history
E. Last meal eaten

Objective assessment

A. Vital signs should be obtained immediately on arrival
   1. Continual noninvasive blood pressure monitoring if available
   2. Do not attempt orthostatic vital signs on unstable patient
B. Baseline assessment of systems
   1. Respiratory
      a) For the patient arriving not intubated
         (1) Patency of airway
         (2) Respiratory effort, pattern, and quality of ventilations
         (3) Bilateral breath sounds
         (4) Position of trachea
      b) For the patient arriving intubated
         (1) Breath sounds with assisted ventilation
         (2) Position and security of tube
         (3) Ease of ventilation
   2. Cardiovascular
      a) Cardiac monitoring for rate and rhythm
      b) Obvious sources of bleeding
      c) Location and description of wound sites
      d) Peripheral pulses distal to injuries
      e) Skin color and temperature
      f) Neck vein distention
      g) Documentation of amount of intravenous fluids infused before patient's arrival in emergency department
   3. Neurological
      a) Cervical, thoracic, and lumbar spine immobilization (assume injury until clinically or radiographically ruled out)
      b) Level of consciousness and mental status
      c) Gross neurological motor or sensory deficits
      d) Pupil size and reactivity
      e) Glasgow Coma Scale
C. Secondary assessment
   1. Monitor vital signs
   2. Observe level of consciousness
   3. Inspect body for obvious deformities caused by trauma
   4. Palpate chest for tenderness, pain, crepitation
   5. Inspect abdomen for trauma, auscultate for bowel sounds
   6. Inspect genitalia for bleeding or hematoma
   7. Inspect extremities for trauma; palpate distal pulses of an injured extremity

POSSIBLE NURSING DIAGNOSES/ANALYSIS

I. Airway clearance, ineffective
II. Anxiety
III. Breathing pattern, ineffective
IV. Cardiac output, alteration in: decreased
V. Comfort, alteration in: pain
VI. Communication, impaired: verbal
VII. Fluid volume deficit: actual and potential
VIII. Grieving, anticipatory
IX. Gas exchange, impaired
X. Tissue perfusion, alteration in: cerebral, cardiopulmonary, peripheral
XI. Skin integrity, impairment of: actual and potential
XII. Urinary elimination: alterations in patterns

PLANNING

I. Preadmission responsibilities based on prehospital notification
   A. Anticipation of need for
      1. Preflushed intravenous lines containing solutions of lactated Ri er's or normal saline for blood transfusion lines
      2. Oxygen and intubation equipment
      3. Trays and equipment for anticipated procedures (refer to app dix A)
      4. Pneumatic antishock trousers on stretcher
   B. Organization of trauma team
      1. Designated "trauma captain"
      2. Assigned tasks to be initiated on patient's arrival
      3. Suggested division for nursing roles (using two nurses)
         a) Primary trauma nurse responsibilities
            (1) Continual patient assessment
            (2) Assisting with procedures
            (3) Direct communication with "trauma captain"
            (4) "Hands-on care"
         b) Secondary trauma nurse responsibilities
            (1) Recording action flow
            (2) Circulating
            (3) Handling initial laboratory specimens
            (4) Telephone communication with blood bank, radiology,

. Priorities for care
  A. Airway management
  B. Spine management
  C. Circulatory management
  D. Immobilization of fractures

. Differential management (because of extensiveness of the differential management, this section is located at the end of the care plan, pp. 238-246)
  A. Categories
    1. Head, neck, and spinal trauma
    2. Chest trauma
    3. Abdominal trauma
    4. Major orthopedic trauma
  B. Descriptions of specific procedures and required equipment are located in appendix A (i.e., supplies and equipment on surgical trays)

IPLEMENTATION

Primary intervention
  A. Initiated simultaneously on patient's arrival
    1. Obtain history from prehospital personnel
    2. Obtain vital signs
    3. Assess airway and ventilate if necessary
    4. Maintain and immobilize spine if indicated
    5. Cut off clothes
  B. Manage airway
    1. Ensure patent airway with adequate ventilations; administer oxygen 4 to 8 L/min via nasal prongs or mask
    2. If inadequate airway or ventilations or patient is unresponsive
      a) Patient arriving intubated
        (1) Designate person to assess quality of breath sounds and determine tube placement
        (2) Assist ventilations with ambu-bag or mechanical ventilator
      b) Patient arriving not intubated
        (1) Suction if indicated
        (2) Ventilate with ambu-bag and mask until airway is controlled
        (3) Method of intubation is determined by physician
          (*a*) Oral route indicated when cervical spine injury not suspected
          (*b*) Nasal route
            i) Indicated with possible cervical spine injury
            ii) Anticipate epistaxis or emesis and prepare suction

c) Cricothyrotomy
(1) Indicated with possible cervical spine injury, unsuccess nasal intubation attempt, or massive facial trauma
(2) (Refer to procedure section in appendix A)
d) Percutaneous transtracheal ventilation
(1) Method of administering high pressure ventilation thro cricothyroid membrane
(2) New approach for trauma patients presently under stud
e) Respiratory compromise because of hemopneumothorax
(1) Indicated by unequal breath sounds or respiratory distr
(2) If patient is in acute distress, chest tube should be inser by physician before x-ray confirmation
(3) (Refer to differential section on chest trauma at the end care plan and the thoracostomy procedure in appendix A
(4) Document type and amount of chest tube drainage

C. Institute cervical spine precautions
1. Align neck with sandbags, secure adhesive tape across forehead cart; place tape across chin to provide additional immobilization; Philadelphia collar along with sandbags and tape to provide best mobilization
2. If patient needs to be moved or is uncooperative, assign someone provide axial traction
3. Obtain portable crosstable lateral cervical x-ray study early in cou of treatment
a) All seven cervical vertebrae should be visualized before x- study is "cleared" by physician
b) Small percentage of fractures are not visualized on lateral view possible, immobilization should not be discontinued until x- series is completed
4. Philadelphia or four-post collar applied by physician in cases of
a) Diagnosed fracture or dislocation
b) Suspected injury not ruled out by x-ray study
c) Uncooperative patient needing more secure immobilization

D. Manage circulation
1. If pulses are absent, continue or initiate CPR; thoracotomy is in cated if there is no response to initial fluid resuscitation; tho cotomy allows for open cardiac massage, relief of tamponade, a aortic cross-clamping for hemorrhage control (refer to proced section in appendix A)

2. Determine initial laboratory data
   a) Obtain hematocrit on patient's arrival
   b) Send blood specimen for type and crossmatch, or if patient is unstable, type specific blood
3. Provide fluid resuscitation based on serial blood pressure and heart rate
   a) Establish large-bore (14 or 16 gauge) intravenous lines with blood administration tubing with lactated Ringer's solution or .9% normal saline
   b) If patient is hypertensive, maintain intravenous line at keep-open rate
   c) Be aware that normotensive patients may be compensating for actual blood loss; continue close observation and frequent vital signs
   d) Respond to hypovolemic shock
      (1) Rapidly infuse fluids, preferably warm fluids; use pressure bags
      (2) Indication for one or two cutdown insertions in saphenous vein (refer to procedure section in appendix A)
      (3) Insert central line to monitor serial CVP readings as indicator of fluid status (refer to procedure section in appendix A)
      (4) Pediatric patients should be given lactated Ringer's or 5% dextrose and normal saline at 20 ml/kg bolus, then titrated to blood pressure
      (5) Blood products or expanders should be given if blood pressure has not stabilized after 2 to 3 liters of fluid or 50 ml/kg
         (*a*) O negative or positive blood should be given only in large acute bleeding with imminent exsanguination such as trauma arrest; its administration complicates further crossmatching
         (*b*) Type-specific blood should be available within 10 to 15 minutes; this is preferred blood for critical patients
         (*c*) Crossmatched blood generally takes 45 to 60 minutes; use for subsequent transfusions such as in the operating room or intensive care unit (ICU)
         (*d*) Autotransfusion procedure may be indicated in trauma facilities equipped to perform this procedure
4. Generally use pneumatic antishock trousers for blood pressure less than 80 mm Hg systolic

5. Consider neurogenic or spinal shock in patients who are hypote sive with normal or decreased heart rates and without a source bleeding; may need to be treated with vasopressor; hypovolem must always be ruled out and corrected first; many young, co ditioned athletes, older patients on beta-blocking agents, or into cated patients will be bradycardic with hypovolemia rather th tachycardic
6. Pericardiocentesis is indicated when pericardial tamponade is su pected (hypotension, elevated CVP, pulsus paradoxus) (refer procedure section in appendix A)
7. Peritoneal lavage (refer to procedure section in appendix A) in cated with
   a) Penetrating trauma of the abdomen with peritoneal penetratio patients with gunshot wounds will usually be taken to t operating room without this procedure having been performe
   b) Penetrating trauma of the lower chest, generally if below t nipple line
   c) Blunt trauma with
      (1) Abdominal tenderness
      (2) Altered mental status from head injury, drugs, alcohol, pain from other major injuries
      (3) Spinal cord injury with inability to sense pain
      (4) Unexplained hypotension or tachycardia
8. Insert indwelling urinary catheter in all critical patients and tho requiring peritoneal lavage
   a) Check urine for presence of blood using a dipstick; if positi spin in urine centrifuge for cell count
   b) Note initial and serial urine output (every 30 to 60 mi utes)—desired: 50 ml/hour for adults, 0.5 ml/kg/hour for ch dren
   c) Stable patients with abdominal or back trauma should ha spontaneously voided urine sample checked for blood
9. Insert nasogastric tube in critical patients
   a) Check for presence of blood
   b) Connect to low suction
10. Arrange rapid transport to operating room, if indicated

II. Secondary intervention
   A. Provide for serial assessment of
      1. Vital signs
      2. Neurological status

3. Fluid status: intravenous infusion, urine output, central venous pressure

B. Additional radiographic and diagnostic procedures should be arranged by trauma team as indicated; for example, intravenous pyelogram, CAT scan, arteriography, tomograms

C. Arrange for 12-lead ECG (indicated with chest trauma)

D. Treat extremity fractures (refer to Chapter 36, Care Plan for Orthopedic Injuries)
   1. Neurovascular checks of extremity
   2. Splint or support for immobilization

E. Treat surface trauma (refer to Chapter 41, Care Plan for Wound Management)

F. Perform admission laboratory studies, as indicated

G. Offer information and support to patient, family, and friends

H. Collect evidence for law enforcement agencies
   1. When removing clothes, avoid cutting through gunshot holes; the material will be examined for powder
   2. Place clothes in paper, NOT PLASTIC, bags
   3. Cover patient's hands with small paper bags if trauma has resulted from gunshot wounds to preserve evidence of powder
   4. Pass on to authorities weapons, bullets, clothes, and other valuables according to policy for maintaining chain of evidence

EVALUATION

I. Patient outcomes/criteria
   A. Patent airway without respiratory distress
   B. Vital signs within normal limits
   C. Improvement or stability of neurological status
   D. Appropriate disposition expeditiously planned: operating room, intensive care unit (ICU), routine admission, emergency department interventions, Emergency Medical Services (EMS) Acute Observation Unit, or home

II. Document initial assessment data, emergency department interventions, and the patient's response to treatment

III. If previous patient outcomes are not reached, the emergency nurse should reevaluate the interventions and change the plan of care accordingly

IV. Perform informal trauma team critique whenever possible
   A. Accurate triage and response of team members
   B. Adequate preparation and availability of supplies
   C. Effective teamwork throughout resuscitation

DISPOSITION

I. Admission criteria
   A. Patients requiring operative intervention
   B. Patients requiring ventilatory management
   C. Patients with unstable vital signs or altered mental status
   D. Patients requiring continuous assessment of injuries or potential injuries
   E. Patients with multiple or major injuries

II. Emergency Medical Services Acute Observation Unit may be appropriate for patients requiring short-term management
   A. Patients after peritoneal lavage with normal studies
   B. Patients requiring repeat chest x-ray studies to observe for development of hemopneumothorax
   C. Patients with mild altered mental status
   D. Patients requiring serial vital signs, repeat hematocrits, and assessment to identify developing complications

III. Discharge guidelines
   A. Provide instructions to patient and family on
      1. Care of surface trauma
      2. Criteria indicating need to return to emergency department
      3. Medications
      4. Injuries resulting from the trauma
   B. Arrange follow-up care if indicated

Injury	Clinical Assessment	Management
HEAD TRAUMA		
Skull Fracture	Obvious open fracture, skull depression, hematoma, developing signs of basilar skull fracture: Battle's sign—mastoid ecchymosis Hemotympanum or bloody drainage from ear "Raccoon" sign—periorbital ecchymosis Otorrhea, rhinorrhea	Confirm with x-ray study (basilar skull fracture often clinical diagnosis and not evident on x ray); open fractures with elevation of fragments are treated in the operating room; also treat with antibiotics; treat altered mental status as ordered with hyperventilation, steroids, diuretics, mannitol; neurosurgical consult may be necessary

jury	Clinical Assessment	Management
tracranial emorrhage Hematoma	Indications of increased intracranial pressure, such as decreased level of consciousness; changes in vital signs: hyperthermia, bradycardia, hypertension, change in respiratory pattern, pupillary changes	Provide intubation, hyperventilation, and oxygenation (hypoxemia, hypercarbia, and acidosis aggravate increased intracranial pressure); restrict fluids unless patient is hypovolemic because of other trauma; administer medications in attempt to decrease cerebral edema: 1. Steroid: dexamethasone for mass lesion 2. Diuretic: furosemide, mannitol Rule out other causes of altered mental status, perform ethanol and toxicology screens; check electrolytes and glucose (refer to Chapter 27, Care Plan for Unresponsive Patient); obtain skull x-ray study and CT scan; neurosurgical consult may be necessary
oncussion	History of trauma with transient loss of consciousness; occasionally no documented loss of consciousness but mild disorientation, irritability, or other nonfocal neurological impairment may be evident; patient may be disoriented or lethargic	Depends on patient's condition and other injuries; patient is usually discharged with head injury instructions; postconcussion syndrome is characterized by headache, dizziness, vertigo, anxiety, and fatigue; may persist for several weeks: treat with aspirin, acetaminophen, prostaglandin inhibitors, phenytoin

Injury	Clinical Assessment	Management
SPINAL AND NECK TRAUMA		
Spinal Cord Injury	Tenderness with palpation of spine, motor or sensory deficits, altered respiratory function with cervical injury 1. C5 or above: apneic 2. Below C5: diaphragmatic breathing Absence of rectal sphincter tone, priapism; may be complicated by spinal shock: hypotension without blood loss, bradycardia, urinary retention, paralytic ileus	Confirm by x-ray study; immobilize cervical spine wi tape and sandbags; keep patient flat on stretcher wi appropriate restraints; assis ventilation as required; consider other causes of hypotension; treat spinal shock with pneumatic anti shock trousers, Trendelenburg position, vasopressor (refer to Chapter 38, Care Plan for Spinal Injury)
Tracheal or Laryngeal Injury	Clinical signs include hoarseness, stridor, dysphonia, dysphagia, dyspnea, neck tenderness, subcutaneous emphysema, soft tissue swelling, loss of normal landmarks	Perform neck and chest x-ra studies, including soft tissu views; intubate or perform cricothyrotomy with ventilatory assistance as neces sary; provide continuous observation
Vascular Injury	Penetrating wound with greater than normal blood loss for wound of similar size; expanding hematoma indicated by airway compression and tracheal deviation; bruits; difference in bilateral pulses and blood pressures taken on carotid artery; neurological deficit (compromised cerebral circulation); hypotension; tachycardia	Perform intubation and venti tion as required; treat hypovolemia and control local bleeding; surgical exploration of selected pe trating wounds may be ne essary; may require angiog raphy
Esophageal or Pharyngeal Injury	Severe pain in throat; dysphagia; in case of esophageal rupture, mediastinal emphysema and subcutaneous emphysema	Diagnose with esophogram o esophagoscopy; administer antibiotics; for rupture, stabilize patient and transport to operating room

jury	Clinical Assessment	Management
HEST TRAUMA		
yocardial ontusion	Anterior chest discomfort, tachycardia, and other dysrhythmias; ST and T waves changes (may occur late or not at all); dyspnea; hypotension; contusion or abrasion over sternum may be present	Treat as myocardial infarction with oxygen, ECG monitor, serial cardiac enzymes, analgesia, and antidysrhythmics as required (refer to Care Plans for Chapter 4, Chest Pain and Chapter 17, Medical Cardiopulmonary Arrest)
ardiac amponade	Symptoms include tachycardia, hypotension, elevated CVP, dyspnea, cyanosis, distended neck veins, distant heart sounds (muffled), pulsus paradoxus	Perform pericardiocentesis (diagnostic and therapeutic); emergency department thoracotomy may be necessary if patient experiences cardiac arrest or is in profound shock; ultimately the patient may go to the operating room
enetrating Vounds to the leart	Myocardial rupture, characterized by: hypotension/tachycardia with rapid exsanguination, decreased ECG voltage, distant heart sounds Valvular rupture, characterized by: chest pain, dyspnea, congestive failure, pulmonary edema, murmur, hemoptysis, hypotension/tachycardia; will occur most often as tamponade	Provide life-support and resuscitative measures for both myocardial and valvular rupture; probably thoracotomy in the emergency department (refer to appendix A for procedure and equipment)
njury to Great 'essels	Mediastinal widening, absent/delayed femoral pulse; patient can have difference in bilateral blood pressure, hypotension/tachycardia; patient may exsanguinate rapidly	Provide fluid resuscitation, life support, thoracotomy as necessary (refer to appendix A for procedure and equipment); angiogram is diagnostic if patient is stable; stabilize patient for transport to operating room
ulmonary Contusion	Tachypnea, dyspnea, hemoptysis, inability to cough, infiltrate on x-ray study	Avoid overhydration; patient may require ventilatory support, antibiotics

Injury	Clinical Assessment	Management
Pneumothorax		
Simple	Sharp pleuritic pain, dyspnea, tachypnea, diminished breath sounds, hyperresonance with percussion, subcutaneous emphysema	Chest x-ray study is diagnost but should not cause dela of treatment when patient exhibits respiratory distres perform thoracostomy (refer to appendix A for procedure and equipment)
Tension	In addition to the above symptoms, there is mediastinal shift and deviated trachea toward unaffected side, distant heart sounds, paradoxical chest-wall movement, distended neck veins, cyanosis	Perform thoracostomy (refer to appendix A for procedure and equipment); man age fluids
Penetrating chest wound	Sucking sound or bubbling at wound site	Use occlusive dressing (vaseline gauze); be alert to sig of developing tension pneumothorax; perform thoracostomy (refer to appendix A for procedure an equipment)
Hemothorax	Signs of pneumothorax and possibly hypotension, tachycardia, and dullness with percussion	Perform thoracostomy (refer to appendix A for procedu and equipment); treat hyp volemia; transport patient to operating room if rapid bleeding continues
Tracheo-bronchial Injury (tear)	Mediastinal and subcutaneous emphysema, dyspnea, and hemoptysis; crunching sound with heartbeat; patient may develop pneumothorax	Perform intubation or cricothyrotomy as indicated; thoracostomy (refer to appendix A for procedure an equipment); diagnosis by bronchoscopy; surgical repair indicated with large tears
Flail Chest	Paradoxical chest motion: flail segment moves inward with inspiration, outward with expiration; tachypnea; dyspnea; cyanosis; possible concomitant injury: hemopneumothorax, myocardial or pulmonary contusion	Perform positive pressure ve tilation (not always used with isolated chest injury); may turn patient to affecte side; manage fluids

ury	Clinical Assessment	Management
b Fracture	Localized pain at site of injury; increased pain with inspiration, movement, cough; splinting or protective posture; patient may have subcutaneous emphysema if complicated by pneumothorax; may develop hemopneumothorax or atelectasis and pneumonia because of pain and splinting	Diagnose by x-ray study and palpation 1. Simple fractures treated with rest, analgesia, intercostal nerve block, and heat 2. Multiple or displaced fractures and injuries in the elderly or debilitated may need observation in the hospital (NOTE: With first-rib fracture, look for fractured clavicle or scapula or injury to esophagus, tracheobronchial tree, or great vessels; lower rib fractures may result in liver or spleen lacerations
ernal racture	Possible associated injuries: myocardial contusion, vascular injury, fractured ribs	Diagnose by lateral chest x-ray study; treat simple fracture with rest and analgesia
iaphragmatic jury	Referred pain to shoulder, dyspnea, hypotension if abdominal viscera compressing heart; penetrating wound as high as fourth intercostal space on level of diaphragm on expiration; penetrating abdominal wound	Perform intubation if clinically indicated; manage fluids; perform gastric decompression and chest x-ray study, which may show abdominal viscera in chest cavity; perform peritoneal lavage, stabilize patient for transport to surgery
BDOMINAL TRAUMA		
epatic Injury ncluding allbladder nd bile ucts)	Right upper quadrant pain with referred pain to shoulder; abdominal tenderness and rigidity may be early peritonitis from blood and bile leaking into peritoneal cavity; hypotension and tachycardia indicative of hypovolemia	1. General management for abdominal trauma: treat hypovolemia; perform peritoneal lavage as diagnostic procedure to detect intraperitoneal bleeding 2. Stab wounds usually are locally explored, followed by peritoneal lavage if penetration is suspected 3. Gunshot wounds are usually explored in the operating room

Injury	Clinical Assessment	Management
Splenic Injury	Left upper quadrant pain and shoulder or scapular pain (Kehr's sign caused by diaphragmatic irritation by blood in peritoneal cavity); local peritoneal irritation; hypotension and tachycardia indicative of hypovolemia; late signs include increased white blood count, progression of pain, absent bowel sounds (NOTE: Subcapsular bleeding may yield negative peritoneal lavage; continued pain and falling hematocrit in patient with tender abdomen may indicate need for scan or ultrasound; observe for delayed rupture; possible associated injuries include left rib fractures or left hemopneumothorax)	(Treatment same as for hepatic injury, p. 243)
Pancreatic Injury	Epigastric pain and guarding; hypotension and tachycardia indicative of hypovolemia; elevated amylase in peritoneal lavage fluid or rising serum or urine amylase levels may not be evident on initial evaluation	(Treatment same as above)
Gastrointestinal Injury	Blood in nasogastric aspirate or stool; hypotension and tachycardia indicative of hypovolemia; perforated viscus usually is associated with pain and diffuse tenderness with peritoneal signs	(Treatment same as above)
Bladder and Urethral Injury	Blood at meatus, dysuria, hematuria, inability to void	If blood is noted at urethral meatus, do not attempt to insert catheter; diagnose by retrograde cystogram or urethrogram

ury	Clinical Assessment	Management
nal Injury	Hematuria; flank pain with or without ecchymosis or mass; pain in upper abdominal quadrant or costovertebral angles; hypotension and tachycardia indicative of hypovolemia	Treat hypovolemia; obtain intravenous pyelogram
DOMINAL TRAUMA IN THE PREGNANT PATIENT		
rtial or mplete acental paration; pture of avid Uterus	Hypotension and tachycardia: because blood volume is increased during pregnancy, as much as 35% may be lost before these signs are manifest; loss is at expense of fetal circulation	Perform fluid resuscitation; may be able to use only leg compartments on pneumatic antishock trousers; do not give oxytoxic drugs or vasopressors (decreases fetal perfusion)
netrating jury of avid Uterus d Fetus	Vaginal bleeding; amniotic fluid leakage; abdominal pain; uterine contractions (NOTE: Abruptio placentae can occur as a result of maternal hypotension unrelated to specific in utero injury; signs of fetal distress: fetal bradycardia—less than 110/min—indicates hypoxia and decreased uterine blood flow; lack of fetal movement)	Third trimester: lateral position with legs elevated to relieve or avoid vena cava compression; perform peritoneal lavage via supraumbilical approach; arrange obstetrical consult for possible C-section
AJOR ORTHOPEDIC TRAUMA		
lvic Fracture	Pain with compression of iliac crest, weight-bearing, or range of motion; patient may have instability of pelvis with palpation; hypotension and tachycardia indicative of blood loss; life-threatening retroperitoneal hemorrhage may occur	Treat hypovolemia; perform x-ray studies to confirm fracture, peritoneal lavage to rule out intraabdominal injuries

Injury	Clinical Assessment	Management
Femur Fracture	Pain with movement; swelling of thigh/hematoma (patient can lose 1-2 units blood into soft tissue); rotation and shortening of extremity because of muscle spasm; hypotension and tachycardia indicative of hypovolemia; compromise to neurovascular status of extremity	Perform fluid resuscitation; splint leg; arrange orthopedic consult for definitive treatment; continue neurovascular checks
Hip Dislocation	Pain, flexion, and most commonly internal rotation	Perform prompt reduction; th longer the hip is dislocated the more likely aseptic necrosis is to develop
Traumatic Amputation	Obvious total or partial amputation of extremity or digit; hypotension and tachycardia if significant blood loss	Perform fluid resuscitation; control bleeding at site Preservation of amputated pa place amputated part in container, wrapping it in a gauze soaked in normal saline; surround container with ice; do not allow contact of ice and skin; do not use dry ice; do not freeze c totally submerge tissue; prepare patient for surgery

CHAPTER 35

NEAR DROWNING

IMPLICATIONS FOR ACTION

Submersion in water for a period of time is known as near drowning. The patient may have a wide variety of clinical problems ranging from mild respiratory distress, hypothermia, and cardiac arrest. The patient may also be lethargic, combative, confused, disoriented, or semicomatose depending on the degree of hypoxemia.

The three priorities for the emergency nurse in caring for these victims are:

1. Maintain a patent airway with adequate ventilation and circulation
2. Treat hypoxia
3. Protect the cervical spine

ASSESSMENT

I. Initial observation
  A. Respiratory status
  B. Level of consciousness
II. Subjective assessment
  A. History of drowning episode
    1. Circumstances via witness account if possible
    2. Water temperature
    3. Type of water (fresh, salt, or contaminated)
    4. Cause of exposure, such as alcohol, drugs, inability to swim
    5. Length of immersion
    6. Hyperventilation before underwater swimming
    7. Any on-the-scene treatment
  B. History of additional trauma (diving accident, cervical spine injury, concussions, skull fracture)
  C. Pertinent medical history
    1. Chronic disease (seizures, cardiovascular compromise, asthma, emphysema)

2. Recent history of respiratory illness (pneumonia, cold)
3. Suicidal ideation
4. Medications
5. Allergies

D. Nonaccidental childhood trauma
E. Associated symptoms: chest pain

III. Objective assessment
A. Complete vital signs
1. Rectal temperature will alert to concurrent hypothermia; howeve it is often elevated
2. Tachycardia may be present
B. Respiratory status
1. Patency of airway
2. Respiratory effort: pattern and quality of ventilations (dyspnea wheezing, cough)
3. Breath sounds: rales, rhonchi
C. Level of consciousness will vary: confusion, irritability, restlessness lethargy, seizures, or coma
D. Cardiovascular status: shock is uncommon in near drowning; if present it is usually the result of an underlying cause such as hypovolemia hypoxia, neurogenic factors, or other concomitant injuries
E. Muscle activity: increased muscle tone

POSSIBLE NURSING DIAGNOSES/ANALYSIS

I. Anxiety
II. Airway clearance, ineffective
III. Breathing pattern, ineffective
IV. Gas exchange, impaired
V. Knowledge deficit (of water hazards)
VI. Tissue perfusion, alteration in: cerebral, cardiopulmonary, renal

PLANNING

I. Priorities for care
A. Promoting adequate ventilation and circulation
B. Preventing complications
C. Decreasing the victim's anxiety
II. Types of drowning
A. Wet: indicates that aspiration has occurred
B. Dry: refers to asphyxia as a result of laryngospasm occurring in absence of aspiration of water
III. Differential management

use	Clinical Assessment	Management
ESH WATER ASPIRATION*		
	(Hypotonic fluid is absorbed rapidly (3-4 min) into the patient's circulation but changes the surface tension characteristics of pulmonary surfactant; consequently the surfactant, when compressed, does not develop sufficient minimal surface tension, which leads to alveolar collapse, intrapulmonary shunting, and hypoxemia) Blood pressure will be elevated; all serum electrolytes except potassium are decreased; chest x-ray study will reveal atelectasis	Provide hyperventilation
ALT WATER ASPIRATION*		
	(Hypertonic fluid draws plasma from circulation into the lungs, producing fluid-filled but perfused alveoli leading to intrapulmonary shunting and hypoxemia) Hypotension, tachycardia; all serum electrolyte levels are elevated; chest x-ray study will reveal haziness	Provide intermittent positive pressure breathing or PEEP

n both types of aspiration there is increased pulmonary resistance and decreased lung comliance, pulmonary edema is common, and large ingestions may cause lethargy, drowsiness, and oma.

MPLEMENTATION

. Primary intervention
   A. Respiratory (oxygen regulated according to arterial blood gases)
      1. For respiratory insufficiency: intubate and give 100% oxygen with positive pressure ventilation
      2. For patients with adequate ventilations, use tight-fitting mask (nonrebreather)

B. Cardiovascular
   1. Maintain CPR on all patients who have been submerged for an extended period—until their temperature is above 32 degrees C (89. degrees F) (refer to Chapter 15, Care Plan for Hypothermia)
   2. ECG monitoring: observe for any rhythm suggestive of hypoxemia
C. Obtain intravenous access
   1. Fresh water aspiration: use dextrose 5%
   2. Salt water aspiration: use lactated Ringer's solution
D. Use central venous pressure monitor and indwelling urinary catheter
E. Maintain cervical spine immobilization until spine is found to be intac (refer to Care Plans for Chapter 34, Major Multiple Trauma and Chapte 38, Spinal Injury)
F. Insert nasogastric tube if there is vomiting or gastric distention
G. Rewarm according to Chapter 15, Care Plan for Hypothermia if patient' core temperature warrants

II. Secondary intervention
   A. Perform laboratory studies
      1. Baseline: arterial blood gases (ABGs), electrolytes, BUN, glucose complete blood count, PT and PTT
      2. Others as indicated: alcohol and drug screens
      3. Chest and cervical spine x-ray studies
   B. Perform serial monitoring of respiratory status, level of consciousness vital signs, urinary output
   C. Administer medications as indicated
      1. Sodium bicarbonate: 0.5 mEq/kg body weight to correct metabolic acidosis
      2. Aminophylline (considered for improvement of bronchodilation)
      3. Isoproterenol via aerosol for bronchospasms
   D. Provide psychological support as appropriate

EVALUATION

I. Patient outcomes/criteria
   A. Improved respiratory status
   B. Improved neurological status
   C. Fluid balance stabilized
   D. Electrolytes within normal limits
II. Document initial assessment data, emergency department interventions and the patient's response to treatment
III. If previous patient outcomes are not reached, the emergency nurse should reevaluate the interventions and change the plan of care accordingly

POSITION

Admission criteria

A. Patients with the following abnormalities should be observed for 12 to 24 hours
   1. Altered mental status
   2. Abnormal chest x-ray study
   3. Abnormal ABGs

Discharge guidelines

A. Discharge reliable asymptomatic patients with normal ABGs and chest x-ray studies after 4-6 hours of observation
B. Teach patient to focus on
   1. Need to return for any pulmonary complications
   2. The dangers of accidental near drownings per geographic area

CHAPTER 36

ORTHOPEDIC INJURIES

IMPLICATIONS FOR ACTION

Patients with orthopedic injuries account for a significant portion of eme gency department visits. The emergency nursing care rendered these patien often affects the therapeutic result these patients achieve. Many times patien who sustain orthopedic injuries also suffer from multiple system injuries as result of major trauma. Following prompt evaluation and treatment of lif threatening injuries or vital function impairment, attention should be directe toward the orthopedic injury.

Major orthopedic injuries of pelvic fracture, femur fracture, hip disloc tion, and traumatic amputation are covered in Chapter 34, Care Plan for Maj Multiple Trauma.

ASSESSMENT

I. Initial observation
  A. Deformity, limb position
  B. Color: erythema, ecchymosis, cyanosis
  C. Skin temperature
  D. Circulation: check color and pulses of extremity
    1. Upper extremity (brachial, radial, ulnar pulses, capillary refill)
    2. Lower extremity (femoral, popliteal, posterior tibial, dorsalis ped pulses)

II. Subjective assessment
  A. History of event producing injury
    1. Mechanism and circumstances surrounding injury, time of occu rence
    2. Prehospital measures to relieve pain or swelling
    3. Range of motion before the accident
    4. Ability to bear weight
    5. Swelling: immediate, delayed, absent
    6. Factors that increase or decrease pain

B. Chief complaint
   1. Localization of pain
   2. Alterations of sensation or movement
C. Pertinent medical history
   1. Any pulmonary problems, bleeding disorders, diabetes
   2. Medications, allergies, immunization status
D. If pediatric patient or patient's family cannot explain how fracture occurred or mechanism of injury, consider possibility of child abuse
E. Be alert to possibility of hip and pelvic fractures in elderly female patients who have even minor falls

Objective assessment

A. Vital signs
B. Level of consciousness (deterioration may signal more severe injury)
C. Point tenderness or pain
D. Mobility: can patient move extremity?
   1. Flexion, extension
   2. Abduction, adduction
   3. Rotation
E. Sensation: paresthesia, hypersthesia, anesthesia (check both distal and proximal to injury site)
F. If open injury, evaluate depth of wound
G. Appearance
   1. Deformity
   2. Dislocation
H. Palpate for any crepitation; do not elicit by moving the fracture
I. Gently handle the pediatric patient since a child may react to a strange environment as well as to the injury itself

OSSIBLE NURSING DIAGNOSES/ANALYSIS

I. Activity intolerance
II. Anxiety
III. Comfort, alteration in: pain
IV. Knowledge deficit (about preventing injuries)
V. Mobility, impaired physical
VI. Self-care deficit: feeding, bathing/hygiene, dressing/grooming, toileting
VII. Skin integrity, impairment of: actual
VIII. Tissue perfusion, alteration in: peripheral

PLANNING

I. Priorities for care
   A. Prevention of further damage or loss of function by
      1. Immobilization
      2. Elevation
   B. Pain control
   C. Isolation of injury if it is not readily apparent
II. Types of injuries
   A. Soft tissue injury: should be considered if there is swelling, ecchymos[is], breaks in skin integrity, and if change in skin temperature exists
III. Differential management

Type of Injury	Clinical Assessment	Management
GENERAL ORTHOPEDIC INJURIES		
Strain	(Occurs to muscle attachments of bone); results from pulling trauma to muscle from overexertion; most commonly occurs in back and arms	Provide rest, immobilization, ice, and elevation
Sprain	(Occurs to ligamentous attachments to joints); an incomplete tearing of the joint capsule and ligaments by forcing beyond the range of the joint; most commonly occurs in ankle and knee	(Treatment same as above)
Tendonitis	(Painful, inflammatory condition at tendinous insertion into bone, occurs especially with range of movement [ROM]); result of overuse; common sites are rotator cuff of shoulder, Achilles tendon, radial aspect of wrist	Provide rest, cold packs, anti-inflammatory measures at site with anesthetic or corticosteroids
Bursitis	(Inflammation of bursa); tenderness, swelling, warmth, redness; common sites: olecranon, greater trochanter of femur, knee	(Treatment same as above)

pe of Injury	Clinical Assessment	Management
ıbluxation	(Loss of continuity between two articular surfaces)	(Treatment described under specific injury)
ıslocation	(Separation of joint surfaces from joint capsule and ligament injury resulting in abnormal location of bones); may be accompanied by fractures; characterized by severe pain, inability to move, and deformity; most commonly occurs in shoulder	(Treatment described under specific injury)
'acture	(Break in continuity of bone or cartilage)	(Treatment described under specific injury)
Closed	(Skin and soft tissue overlying fracture site are intact)	(Treatment described under specific injury)
Open	(Fracture communicates with a break in the skin)	(Treatment described under specific injury)
'ECIFIC ORTHOPEDIC INJURIES		
pper Extremity		
Acromioclavicular (AC) separation	Resulting from fall on point of shoulder; patient is unable to raise arm or bring it across chest	Treat with immobilization (sling and swath); definitive treatment of complete (third-degree) separation is surgical repair and 6 weeks in a shoulder immobilizer
Shoulder dislocation	Characterized by severe pain, inability to move, and deformity; 95% are anterior, frequently from fall on extended arm that has been abducted and externally rotated; posterior dislocation occurs when arm is abducted and internally rotated, as in seizure activity	Perform neurovascular assessment; often decreased sensation over shoulder; intervene immediately; treatment is closed reduction with sling and swath; dislocation is often recurrent and may require eventual surgical intervention; administer intravenous analgesics and muscle relaxants

Type of Injury	Clinical Assessment	Management
Clavicular fracture	Most common fracture of childhood, usually caused by fall on outstretched hand; point tenderness, deformity along clavicular line, swelling, crepitus; patient will support injured arm with unaffected arm; child will refuse to raise affected arm	Vascular checks on ulna and radial pulses are imperativ treatment involves reduction of fracture and immobilization with figure eight wrap
Humeral fracture	Patient has pain and is unable to move arm; ecchymosis evident on axillary aspect of arm or thoracic wall; severance of radial nerve is evidenced by numbness of thumb and immediate inability of patient to raise hand at wrist	Temporarily immobilize the arm with a figure eight wrap; apply cold packs; sling or splint; arrange orthopedic consult for definitive care
Elbow fracture	Patient has severe pain, tenderness, and rapid swelling; arm has distorted appearance and cannot be flexed; patient usually supports arm in flexed position Volkman's contracture: complication of elbow injury occurring within 48 hours; constant burning pain in forearm, swollen and cyanotic hands and fingers, radial pulse absent, numbness in fingers and thumb, pain in extending fingers	Perform immediate and continuous neurovascular assessment; immobilize arm; apply ice packs to reduce edema; surgical interventic may be required
Radius and ulnar fractures	Patient has point tenderness, swelling, deformity	Assess neurovascular status; splint to immobilize; apply cold packs; arrange orthopedic consult for definitive care

pe of Injury	Clinical Assessment	Management
rist racture	Occurs most frequently in elderly; patient has pain, swelling, point tenderness, deformity; in children, Colles fracture will often become apparent only 2-3 days later because of minimal swelling	Splint limb in presenting position; apply cold packs and elevate; arrange orthopedic consult for definitive care
Hand and inger fractures	Pain, swelling, deformity, inability to use hand	Assess neurovascular status; splint fracture in functional position; apply cold packs; arrange orthopedic consult for definitive care
wer Extremity		
Pelvic racture	(See Chapter 34, Care Plan for Major Multiple Trauma)	
Hip dislocation	(See Chapter 34, Care Plan for Major Multiple Trauma)	
Hip fracture	Deformity, local swelling, point tenderness; variable degrees of extremity shortening and external rotation; inability to bear weight	Immobilize; provide intravenous access; arrange for eventual surgical intervention
Femur fracture	(See Chapter 34, Care Plan for Major Multiple Trauma)	
Knee fracture	Severe pain, point tenderness, inability to walk, swelling, inability to straighten leg	Avoid manipulation; apply cold packs; place patient in supine resting position; arrange orthopedic consult for definitive care
Tibia and fibula fractures	Severe pain, inability to dorsiflex foot; capillary return to toes may be diminished	Immobilize and elevate; apply cold packs; arrange orthopedic consult for definitive care
Ankle fracture	Patient has immediate pain, swelling, immobility, and inability to bear weight; also point tenderness, deformity	Immobilize, apply cold packs, elevate; arrange orthopedic consult for definitive care

Type of Injury	Clinical Assessment	Management
Foot fracture	Severe pain, deformity; patient tends to throw foot outward	Apply cold packs, elevate; arrange orthopedic consult for definitive care
Amputation		
Extremity	(See Chapter 34, Care Plan for Major Multiple Trauma)	
Digit	(See Chapter 41, Care Plan for Wound Management)	
Compartment Syndrome	Intense localized pain with ROM; pain is unaffected by elevation, immobilization, or anesthesia; decreased sensation; pulse will be present even with severe compartment ischemia	Elevate and provide analgesia; physician may perform emergency fasciotomy

IMPLEMENTATION

I. Primary intervention
  A. Follow guidelines in differential management section
  B. Immobilize affected area
    1. Splinting of joint above and below area of involvement
    2. Sling
    3. Pillows
    4. Sandbags, blanket rolls
  C. Elevation
  D. Cold packs to extremity
  E. Order x-ray studies after initial assessment
    1. Check with physician if unsure of appropriate views
    2. Patients should have adequate splinting before having x-ray studie
  F. Remove rings from injured hands
  G. Treat open fractures
    1. Check tetanus immunization status (refer to Chapter 41, Care Pla for Wound Management for tetanus schedule)
    2. Anticipate parenteral antibiotics
    3. Care for wound
      a) Culture the wound
      b) Apply pressure dressing for bleeding
      c) Apply sterile dressing with povidone-iodine

. Secondary intervention
  A. Check patient's comfort and safety
    1. Siderails or lap belt
    2. Positioning
    3. Analgesia: give early in emergency department course after injury confirmed
  B. Arrange for family involvement
    1. Keep family informed of progress
    2. Assess learning needs of family and patient for discharge

VALUATION

I. Patient outcomes/criteria
  A. Improvement in pain after medication, cold packs, immobilization
  B. Improved or no further deterioration of neurovascular status
I. Document initial assessment data, emergency department interventions, and patient's response to treatment
I. If previous patient outcomes are not reached, the emergency nurse should reevaluate the interventions and change the plan of care accordingly

ISPOSITION

. Admission criteria
  A. Clavicular fractures with first and second rib involvement
  B. All compartment syndromes or suspected ones
  C. All major orthopedic injuries
. Discharge guidelines
  A. Provide instructions
    1. Elevation and cold packs for 24 hours
    2. Pain medication as ordered
    3. Explanation of aftercare sheets (refer to appendix E, discharge instruction sheets)
      a) Crutches
      b) Cast Care
      c) Sprains and Fractures
  B. Follow-up
    1. Advise patient to come for 24-hour cast check in emergency department
    2. Tell patient to return to emergency department for changes in color or sensation of injured limb
    3. Arrange orthopedic consultation follow-up

CHAPTER 37

SEXUAL ASSAULT

IMPLICATIONS FOR ACTION

Sexual assault and its aftermath is often both a physical and psychologi emergency for the victim. The first priority is to give the patient a private ro and continuous emotional support during assessment and emergency int ventions. If the patient is physically unstable from the trauma associated w rape: assure ABCs, obtain intravenous access, provide oxygen, control ble ing, and immobilize fractures. Once physical stability is assured, a thorou assessment and examination following appropriate state laws for collecting e dence for rape victims can begin. Initially, patients may not want to charges. Assure the patient that collected objective evidence can ONLY obtained immediately following the assault. The ultimate decision will be up the patient as to whether or not to file charges. The following care plan applicable to both female and male victims.

ASSESSMENT

I. Initial observation
  A. Assessment of acute medical condition, life-threatening injuries
  B. Observation of patient's general emotional state on arrival in em gency department
II. Subjective assessment
  A. History of the incident may be obtained by a physician or a nurse (cord patient's own words whenever possible)
    1. Time elapse since assault
    2. Has patient bathed, douched, urinated, defecated, or changed clo ing since incident?
    3. Any evidence of physical violence
      a) Any threats
      b) Use of weapons
    4. Oral, vaginal, anal penetration

B. Pertinent medical history
   1. History of any serious illness, including venereal disease
   2. Date and time of last voluntary sexual intercourse (is patient sexually active?)
   3. Last menstrual period
   4. Type of birth control used, if any
   5. Gravidity and parity
   6. Confirmed pregnancy
   7. Current medications
   8. Allergies
   9. Tetanus status

I. Objective assessment
   A. Complete vital signs: important especially in acute trauma to victim since they will assist in detecting any subtle medical emergencies
   B. Physical injuries
      1. Have patient remove own clothing, if at all possible, and place in a paper, not plastic, bag
      2. Note any bruises, scratches, and other injuries on patient's body

OSSIBLE NURSING DIAGNOSES/ANALYSIS

I. Anxiety
II. Comfort, alteration in: pain
III. Coping, ineffective individual
IV. Fear
V. Grieving, anticipatory
VI. Powerlessness
VII. Self-concept, disturbance in: self-esteem
III. Skin integrity, impairment of: actual and potential
IX. Rape trauma syndrome

LANNING

. Priorities for care
   A. Treatment of life-threatening emergencies
   B. Emotional support for victim
   C. Evidence collection
. Differential management (not applicable)

MPLEMENTATION

. Primary intervention
   A. Stabilize and treat patient for any apparent medical problems before evidence collection examination (refer to other care plans as appropriate)

II. Secondary intervention
   A. Provide emotional support to patient, such as holding hand, talking patient, explaining the process of the evidence examination, and hel ing patient feel as safe as possible
   B. Assist physician with evidence collection examination and place e dence in well-labeled paper, not plastic, containers; comply with coun and state procedures
      1. Collect scrapings from under patient's fingernails
      2. Collect an aspirated or scraped specimen from the patient's orific for sperm as indicated: pharynx, vagina, rectum, urethra; the specimens should also be cultured for gonorrhea; use only water saline on speculum, no lubricants
      3. Comb patient's pubic hair for foreign hair
      4. Pluck a few of the patient's own pubic hairs and head hairs
      5. Draw blood for syphilis testing
      6. Remember to seal and label all specimens; DO NOT leave specime in examination room at any time; make sure evidence is handed ov to appropriate personnel
   C. Administer medications
      1. Tetanus prophylaxis for any open wounds (refer to Chapter 41, Ca Plan for Wound Management for tetanus schedule)
      2. Antibiotics, if wounds are contaminated
      3. Venereal disease prophylaxis if indicated
      4. Pregnancy prophylaxis should be offered by physician—it is a p tient decision: norgestrel 1.5 mg with .05 ethinyl estradiol (Ovral) tablets immediately, 2 tablets in 12 hours
   D. After evidence examination is complete, offer patient a shower, mout wash, change of clothing
   E. Arrange, with patient's permission, follow-up counseling through a ra crisis center

EVALUATION

I. Patient outcomes/criteria
   A. Stabilization of physical status
   B. Stabilization of emotional status once examination is completed
II. Document initial assessment data—using wording of "reported sexual sault" or "patient states was assaulted"—emergency department interve tion, and patient's response to treatment
III. If previous patient outcomes are not reached, the emergency nurse shou reevaluate the interventions and change the plan of care accordingly

SPOSITION

Admission criteria

A. If physical injuries are present, a medical workup is required

B. If emotional status requires precautions against suicidal ideation, etc.

Discharge guidelines

A. Review patient information sheet with patient and family member

B. Encourage follow-up regarding

   1. Laboratory results: venereal disease test results
   2. Counseling: provide list of service agencies available; encourage patient to ventilate feelings and seek assistance in dealing with problems

C. Refer to crisis intervention or social service department for follow-up

CHAPTER 38

SPINAL INJURY

IMPLICATIONS FOR ACTION

This care plan deals with the patient who is suspected of having an isola spinal cord injury (refer to the Care Plan for Multiple Trauma for care of patient with a combination of traumatic injuries).

If a patient has a cervical spinal injury, airway management and immob zation of the spine are equal first priorities. The emergency nurse should sume spinal injury until it's ruled out radiographically. For example, intubat the patient in respiratory failure may be the first procedure performed but without regard to maintaining proper alignment of the spine. As with any cr cally ill patient, life support measures should be instituted before obtainin complete history and physical examination.

ASSESSMENT

I. Initial observation
   A. Respiratory status
   B. Immobilization of spine
   C. Movement of extremities
II. Subjective assessment
   A. History
      1. Mechanism of injury reported by patient or witnesses
      2. Extent of movement and sensation after injury
      3. Method of immobilization at scene
      4. Past injuries to spinal column and residual deficits
   B. Associated symptoms
      1. Complaints of pain along spinal column, with or without palpati
      2. Numbness or tingling of extremities (NOTE: Presence or absenc cervical pain is a reliable indicator only in the alert patient; alw consider spinal injury in the traumatized, unconscious, or int icated patient or when the mechanism of injury is consistent w potential injury)

. Objective assessment
  A. Vital signs (be alert to respiratory distress, hypotension)
  B. Mental status
  C. Ability to move extremities; deficits occur at and distal to the level of injury
  D. Spinal cord injury may be manifested as
    1. Absence of anal sphincter tone
    2. Urinary retention
    3. Loss of sweating reflex
    4. Loss of vasomotor tone
  E. Obvious spinal deformity

)SSIBLE NURSING DIAGNOSES/ANALYSIS

I. Airway clearance, ineffective
II. Anxiety
'II. Bowel elimination, alteration in: incontinence
.V. Breathing pattern, ineffective
V. Comfort, alteration in: pain
VI. Coping, ineffective family: compromised
II. Coping, ineffective individual
II. Grieving, anticipatory
X. Injury: potential for
X. Knowledge deficit (related to injury)
XI. Mobility, impaired physical
II. Self-care deficit: feeding, bathing/hygiene, dressing/grooming, toileting
II. Skin integrity, impairment of: potential
IV. Urinary elimination, alteration in: patterns

.ANNING

Priorities for care
  A. Airway management
  B. Adequate immobilization
  C. Treatment of spinal shock
Differential management

Type of Injury	Clinical Assessment	Management
FRACTURE, DISLOCATION, SUBLUXATION		
	Patient may have fracture of vertebral column without cord injury; edema at site of injury slowly resolves; may result in return of some motor and sensory function; be alert to respiratory compromise in injury above C-5 as a result of paralysis of diaphragm and intercostal muscles	Immobilize; manage airway
NEUROGENIC SHOCK (SPINAL SHOCK)		
	Loss of motor and sensory reflex arcs of vasomotor control; may take weeks or months to resolve; hypotension, bradycardia, urinary and bowel retention	Hypotension usually doesn't respond to fluid challenge; t with vasopressors, pneumati antishock trousers; consider other causes of hypotension
RUPTURED DISK AND COMPRESSION FRACTURE OF VERTEBRAE		
	Compression of nerve roots against vertebrae results in pain in back and extremities distal to injury; muscle spasms; most common causes are auto accidents or falls from a height; may be result of lifting heavy objects or falling on back; usually lumbar, may be thoracic spinal injury	Provide bedrest; traction; antic pate possible surgery; analge
WHIPLASH		
	Sudden hyperextension of neck causing damage to muscles, ligaments, and possibly nervous tissue of cervical spine	Provide rest, heat, analgesia, s collar

IPLEMENTATION

Primary intervention

A. Protect airway and supply oxygen
   1. Nasotracheal intubation preferred to endotracheal intubation to avoid hyperextension of neck
   2. Perform cricothyrotomy if unable to intubate nasotracheally as with massive facial injuries (refer to appendix A for procedure and equipment)
   3. Suction as needed
   4. If patient vomits, log roll to side and suction (requires several people, one responsible for axial traction)

B. Immobilize
   1. Cervical spine
      a) Properly align skull to body
      b) Transport patient only when necessary, on backboard or "scoop" with neck secured; place on hard stretcher, position sandbags on both sides of head, and tape securely across forehead and possibly chin to stretcher
      c) Caution cooperative patient to remain stationary; restrain if necessary
      d) Cut off clothing if necessary; do NOT move patient to remove items
      e) Lateral cervical x-ray study must reveal seven cervical vertebrae to be "cleared"; if patient is unstable, this should begin with a portable lateral cervical spine study and AP thoracic and lumbar studies in the emergency department; complete the series in radiology when patient has been stabilized
      f) Patients who are ambulatory should have the neck immobilized if they exhibit cervical spine pain and should not ambulate until spinal injury has been ruled out
   2. Lower spine injuries
      a) Position patient flat on a stretcher
      b) Patient should not ambulate until spinal injury has been ruled out

C. Treat concomitant injuries as indicated (refer to appropriate care plan)

Secondary intervention

A. If spinal injury is confirmed
   1. Physician will apply stabilizing collar (four-poster or Philadelphia collar) or traction device (Crutchfield tongs, Halo)
   2. Insert indwelling urinary catheter for urinary retention

3. Insert nasogastric tube as paralytic ileus is common with cervical a thoracic spinal injuries
4. Obtain serial vital signs with reevaluation of respiratory status, p tient's ability to move extremities, and level of sensation

B. Be supportive to patient and family; the loss of control that occurs w spinal injuries is very frightening; patients and their families need to educated to the expected plan for the patient and to the fact that p manent residual damage from the injury may not be known for so time

EVALUATION

I. Patient outcomes/criteria
   A. Evidence of no further deterioration of neurological deficit
   B. Vital signs within normal limits
II. Document initial assessment data, emergency department interventio and the patient's response to treatment
III. If previous patient outcomes are not reached, the emergency nurse shou reevaluate the interventions and change the plan of care accordingly

DISPOSITION

I. Admission criteria
   A. Confirmed spinal injury
   B. Patient requiring use of Halo traction, Crutchfield tongs, Stryker fram or fusion of fracture in the operating room
II. Discharge guidelines
   A. Many patients arriving via ambulance with cervical precautions w turn out not to have spinal injury and can be discharged
   B. Recommend rest, heat, and analgesia for muscular injuries
   C. Provide discharge instruction sheets for patients with back injur (refer to appendix E)

CHAPTER 39

SURFACE TRAUMA: BURNS

IMPLICATIONS FOR ACTION

The care plan for surface trauma is covered by this chapter and the two that follow on radioactive contamination and wound management. Management of the patient with major burns requires a coordinated effort among staff with airway management and fluid resuscitation as the initial tasks. Actual burn care given in the emergency department will vary among institutions depending on the availability of a burn unit. If on initial observation of patient or by history the patient is presumed to have a major burn, the emergency nurse should proceed to the implementation section of the care plan. Those interventions are carried out before obtaining a thorough history and physical assessment. Pain medication should be given as soon as possible during treatment of the patient.

Most minor burns can be successfully treated on an outpatient basis with frequent follow-up visits to monitor the healing process.

ASSESSMENT

I. Initial observation
    A. Respiratory status
    B. Extent of burns
    C. Level of consciousness
    D. Color of burned skin
II. Subjective assessment
    A. History of events from patient or witnesses
        1. Type of injury agent (thermal, chemical, electrical)
        2. Duration of exposure
        3. Possibility of concomitant injuries
    B. Past medical history
    C. Allergies and tetanus immunization (refer to Chapter 41, Care Plan for Wound Management, for tetanus schedule)

- D. Degree of pain
- E. Dyspnea

III. Objective assessment
- A. Vital signs
  1. Careful evaluation of respiratory status; skin burns may be accor panied by carbon monoxide or cyanide poisoning caused by t toxic products of combustion
  2. Continuous rectal temperature for extensive burns
- B. Level of consciousness should be checked; burn injury should n cause decreased mentation; assess patient for another cause of neur logical deficit
- C. Peripheral pulses must be monitored with extensive extremity burn check color and characteristics of burned tissue
- D. Estimation of degree and percentage of burns (see tables opposite)

POSSIBLE NURSING DIAGNOSES/ANALYSIS

I. Airway clearance, ineffective
II. Breathing pattern, ineffective
III. Cardiac output, alteration in: decreased
IV. Comfort, alteration in: pain
V. Fluid volume deficit, actual and potential
VI. Gas exchange, impaired
VII. Knowledge deficit (regarding burn risks)
VIII. Nutrition, alteration in: less than body requirements
IX. Skin integrity, impairment of: actual and potential
X. Tissue perfusion, alteration in: cerebral, cardiopulmonary, renal, gastr intestinal, peripheral

PLANNING

I. Priorities for care
- A. Airway management
- B. Fluid management
- C. Burn management
- D. Pain management

II. Differential management (see pp. 272-274)

ule of Nines*

Area	Percentage of Body Surface
Head	9
Right upper extremity (RUE)	9
Left upper extremity (LUE)	9
Right lower extremity (RLE)	18
Left lower extremity (LLE)	18
Anterior trunk	18
Posterior trunk	18
Perineum	1

or adults; not accurate for infants and children.

elative Percentages of Areas Affected by Growth*

	Birth	1 Yr	5 Yr	10 Yr	15 Yr	Adult
alf of head	9 1/2%	8 1/2%	6 1/2%	5 1/2%	4 1/2%	3 1/2%
alf of thigh	2 3/4%	3 1/4%	4%	4 1/4%	4 1/2%	4 3/4%
alf of leg	2 1/2%	2 1/2%	2 3/4%	3%	3 1/4%	3 1/2%

or children, the Lund-Browder Chart makes allowances for the large surface area of certain dy areas (such as the head) in the growing child.

Burns	Clinical Assessment	Management
CLASSIFICATION OF BURNS		
First Degree	Involves only superficial layers of epidermis; skin is erythematous, caused by congestion and vasodilation of intradermal vessels; painful (i.e., sunburn)	Apply room-temperature sterile saline soak if burn occurred recently; cleanse with saline; keep wound clean and dry
Second Degree (partial thickness)	Varying depths of destruction to epidermis with congestion and coagulation present; epithelial regeneration may occur although area is susceptible to infection and may progress to third degree; skin may have blistering with quick capillary refill; if deeper thickness involved, injury will appear white, without blistering and have poor vascularization	Apply room-temperature sterile saline soak if recen injury; cleanse with mild povidone-iodine and consider possible debridemen apply occlusive dressing with silver sulfadiazine or petroleum and bulky bandage
Third Degree (full thickness)	Destruction of all skin elements; may involve damage to underlying tissue (referred to as fourth degree); skin has a yellow-white, leathery, or translucent appearance depending on depth; lack of sensitivity to touch; eschar or constrictive tissue causing venous stasis or obliteration of arterial circulation, as well as ischemic necrosis, may occur	Apply room-temperature sterile saline soak if recen injury; perform povidone-iodine scrub and debridement (may not be started until patient is in burn inpatient unit); escharotomy may be performed
TYPES OF BURNS		
Thermal	Caused by flame or hot liquid (see previous discussion of first-, second-, and third-degree burns)	
Chemical	Burn injury may occur without heat production	Remove clothes; irrigate wit large amounts of cool wat (may require several hours especially for alkaline burr if in eye, use normal saline (see Chapter 31 for specif eye burn management)

urns	Clinical Assessment	Management
PECIFIC CHEMICAL BURNS		
	(Neutralizing agents not indicated for most chemicals except as follows)	
ydrofluoric cid	Released fluoride ions penetrate deeply into skin and remain active until bound with calcium or magnesium; may produce deep burn injury	Irrigate with large amount of water; apply magnesium sulfate paste of hyamen 0.2%; if the burn is caused by greater than 20% hydrofluoric acid, local injection of 10% calcium glucuronate is recommended
hosphorus burns when xposed to air)	Deep tissue injury; site may appear yellowish or necrotic, glows in dark; may be a risk for systemic phosphorus poisoning	Flush with water; cover burn area with moist dressing to avoid air; irrigate wound with 1%-2% copper sulfate solution, then repeat water irrigation
odium and ithium Metal urns	Contact with these metals and water causes release of hydrogen gas	Water irrigation is contraindicated; immerse wound in oil to prevent further combustion; remove remaining particles
henol Carbolic Acid)	(An aromatic hydrocarbon widely used in industry; may produce systemic toxicity as well as a local burn) cardiovascular, metabolic acidosis, CNS stimulation	Flush with water and apply solvent: polyethylene glycol, prophylene glycol glycerol, vegetable oil, or soap and water
ar or Asphalt	Usually splash areas	Immediately cool with water; remove tar with petroleum base ointment such as Neosporin or Polysporin (or mineral oil)
LECTRICAL BURNS		
	Arc type: common cause of mouth and lip burns in children; direct contact burns have entrance and exit points; usually greater tissue damage than is visibly apparent	Perform fluid resuscitation if internal injuries are suspected; locate pathway of conduction; monitor arrhythmias and admit patient for observation

Burns	Clinical Assessment	Management
INHALATION BURNS*		
	Burns to upper airway may lead to obstruction during first 24 hours after contact; check for singed nasal hair, facial burns, blistering, red or dry mucosa, hoarseness, wheezing, tachypnea, soot-stained sputum, cyanosis; circumferential neck burns, oral/pharyngeal burns	Observe for airway edema an prepare for intubation if in dicated; observe for fluid overload with respiratory compromise in isolated respiratory tract burns

*Inhalation of carbon monoxide and toxic products is discussed in Chapter 33, Care Plan for Inhalation Injuries.

IMPLEMENTATION

I. Primary intervention
  A. Manage airway
    1. Facial and respiratory burns may require oral or nasopharyngeal i tubation with assisted ventilation
      a) Indicated for burns to face, decreased or congested brea sounds, difficulty in breathing
    2. Provide humidified oxygen via nasal prongs or mask at 6 to 8 L/mi
    3. If carbon monoxide poisoning is suspected, provide oxygen at 100 by nonrebreather mask
    4. Obtain arterial blood gases
    5. Early intubation and respirator management may be necessary
  B. Manage fluids and monitor cardiovascular status
    1. Provide intravenous management
      a) Indicated for burns involving 10% to 15% surface area or great
      b) Use one or two peripheral large-bore IVs; central line for C measurements
      c) If possible, avoid burned tissue for IV site
      d) Lactated Ringer's solution is the fluid of choice for first 24 hou
      e) Estimated fluid replacement: 2.5 to 4 ml/kg/% of burn over fir 24 hours (adults and children); half of this amount in the first hours
      f) Insert indwelling urinary catheter to monitor urine output; kee at 30 to 50 ml/hour for adults; 1 ml/kg/hour in children

  - *g*) Insert nasogastric tube to treat ileus and to lower risk of burn-induced gastrointestinal bleeding
2. Monitor cardiac activity
   - *a*) Especially important to observe for signs of injury and ectopy with electrical burns
   - *b*) May place electrode on burn tissue if necessary
3. Use warm IV fluids and blankets to prevent hypothermia

C. Provide major burn management
1. Refer to table in differential management section for care of specific types of burns
2. Management of patients with major burns warrants use of sterile masks, gown, and gloves as precaution against infection
3. Remove all the patient's clothing and jewelry
4. Start water irrigation immediately for chemical burns
5. Using sterile technique, cover thermal burns with 4 × 4s (fine mesh gauze or sterile sheets soaked in cool normal saline); do not use iced saline as it may unnecessarily lower body temperature
6. Circumferential burns may cause venous status and obliterate arterial circulation resulting in ischemic necrosis; check peripheral pulses, sensation, and movement on extremity wounds; escharotomy may be performed in the emergency department
7. Perform povidone-iodine scrub and debridement for second- and third-degree burns

D. Provide minor burn care
1. Perform povidone-iodine cleansing with saline rinse
2. Apply thin layer of silver sulfadiazine, cover with fine mesh gauze and rolled stretch gauze
3. Or apply petroleum and rolled stretch gauze

E. Administer medications
1. Give tetanus immunization for extensive burns; give if greater than 10 years for minor burns (refer to Chapter 41, Care Plan for Wound Management for tetanus schedule)
2. Give pain medication
   - *a*) IV: morphine, meperidine are common
   - *b*) IM medications are poorly absorbed with extensive burns

. Secondary intervention

A. Insert nasogastric tube as ileus and gastric dilation are common with extensive burns; patient should remain NPO

B. Rule out other injuries (such as from auto accident, fall, etc.)

C. Perform diagnostic tests
1. Laboratory: complete blood count, electrolytes and glucose, BUN, creatinine PT/PTT, platelet count, arterial blood gases, urinalysis

2. Chest x-ray study, 12-lead ECG
3. Carbon monoxide and cyanide levels if exposure is suspected

D. Provide emotional support to patient and family
E. Evaluate burns of children for possibility of nonaccidental trauma (refe to Care Plan on Child Abuse)
F. Perform continual assessment of vital signs and hydration as evidence by CVP and urine output

EVALUATION

I. Patient outcomes/criteria
   A. Vital signs within normal limits
   B. Absence of respiratory distress
   C. Relief of pain
   D. Adequate hydration evidenced by
      1. Absence of pulmonary edema
      2. Adequate urinary output

II. Document initial assessment data, emergency department intervention and patient's response to treatment

III. If previous patient outcomes are not reached, the emergency nurse shoul reevaluate the interventions and change the plan of care accordingly

DISPOSITION

I. Admission criteria
   A. Any patient with second- or third-degree burns involving face, nec hands, feet, or perineum should be evaluated for possible admission
   B. Patients with second-degree burns of 15% to 25% or more and virtual all those with third-degree burns should be admitted
   C. Patients with electrical burns
   D. Patients with inhalation burns
   E. Any patients with burns caused by nonaccidental trauma
   F. Intensive care unit or burn unit admission depends on the severity c the burn

II. Discharge guidelines
   A. Provide burn care instruction sheet with dressing change informatio (or arrange for patient to return to the emergency department fo changes)
   B. Arrange follow-up wound checks
   C. Give medication instructions
   D. Give prevention instructions as appropriate

HAPTER 40

SURFACE TRAUMA: RADIOACTIVE CONTAMINATION

PLICATIONS FOR ACTION

the patient is seriously injured, emergency life-saving assistance should be en immediately, regardless of real or suspected contamination. Historically radiation accident victim has ever been so contaminated as to present a reat to the care providers. However, contaminated patients ideally should ter the emergency department through a separate, protected entrance. All edical personnel should wear protective, disposable clothing including sur-al gloves and shoe covers (see box at end of chapter).

SESSMENT

. Initial observation
   - A. Determine presence of life-threatening injuries or illness
   - B. Check patient with survey meter (Geiger counter) to determine contamination status
   - C. Determine level of consciousness (early onset of CNS symptoms, including convulsions, usually indicate a massive exposure)

. Subjective assessment
   - A. History of exposure
     1. Exact type: external vs. internal, whole body vs. partial body; (if internal, determine route of entry: inhalation vs. oral ingestion)
     2. Radioactive materials involved
     3. Duration of exposure
   - B. Determine presence of "radiation syndrome": nausea, vomiting, or ataxia

. Objective assessment
   - A. Vital signs: contamination usually does not cause change; if changes occur, look for other injuries or illnesses

B. Presence of injuries such as open wounds that may be contaminate
C. Presence of any neurological findings: disorientation, ataxia, or conv sions

POSSIBLE NURSING DIAGNOSES/ANALYSIS

I. Anxiety
II. Skin integrity, impairment of: potential
III. Comfort, alteration in: pain

PLANNING

I. Priorities for care
   A. Treatment of life-threatening emergencies according to specific etiolo
   B. Decontamination
   C. Fluid management
   D. Pain management
II. Differential management

Degree of Contamination	Clinical Assessment	Management
EXTERNAL CONTAMINATION		
Survival Probable	No initial symptoms or patient may have mild nausea and vomiting; exposure in this group estimated to have been less than 200 rad	Perform serial complete blood counts and observation; admission usually not necessar
Survival Possible	Nausea and vomiting lasting 24 to 48 hours; patient may exhibit thrombocytopenia, granulocytopenia, and lymphopenia; exposure dosage range between 200-800 rad	Provide fluid and electrolyte therapy if vomiting is severe administer antiemetics; provide protective isolation if lymphocyte count at 48 hou is less than 1200
Survival Improbable	Rapid onset of fulminating nausea, vomiting, diarrhea; bone marrow aplasia and pancytopenia; exposure greater than 800 rad; if CNS symptoms are present, it can be assumed that patient has received a large dose	Provide intense fluid and electrolyte therapy; possible bon marrow transplantation; administer analgesia with na cotics and sedatives; offer vigorous supportive therapy; however, prognosis is dismal in mass casualty situations, offer supportive therapy for comfort only

egree of ontamination	Clinical Assessment	Management
TERNAL CONTAMINATION		
	Same as external contamination, corresponds to rad absorbed	Determine exactly what radionucleotides are involved; administration of a blocking or chelating agent, such as Lugol's solution, calcium aiosodium edeta, etc., depends on element involved; use standard measures for ingestion (refer to Chapter 20, Care Plan for Poisoning); all excretions should be saved for proper disposal; for acute inhalation, provide early bronchopulmonary lavage

MPLEMENTATION

. Primary intervention
   A. Assure airway, breathing, and circulation (ABCs)
   B. Provide decontamination
      1. Immediately undress patient and place all clothing in sealed containers labeled "radioactive waste"
      2. Cleanse exposed skin with soap and water and repeat cleansing as many times as necessary, depending on dosimeter readings received
      3. Open wounds have first priority and should be decontaminated by scrubbing with soap and water; apply adhesive surgical drapes and irrigate the wound with copious amounts of saline; frequent monitoring of wound with a Geiger counter will determine when irrigation can be discontinued
         a) Irrigate contaminated eyes with water from medial aspect outward; monitor, survey, and repeat as necessary
         b) Irrigate contaminated ear canals gently and copiously with small amounts of water at a single irrigation to prevent induction of vertigo
         c) Rinse contaminated nares or mouth gently with small amounts of water; turn head to side or down, as patient's condition permits; suction frequently; to prevent water from entering stomach, in-

sert nasogastric tube, suction, and monitor if gastric contents ar contaminated; lavage with small aliquots of normal saline unt contents are cleared of contamination

C. Infuse dextrose 5% and half normal saline or normal saline for orthc stasis and persistent vomiting
D. Administer analgesia for pain via narcotics and sedatives
E. Give antiemetics
F. Obtain laboratory data, including complete blood count and platele count
G. Prevent contamination of self and others by proper disposal of clothing supplies, emesis, secretions, and excretions

II. Secondary intervention
A. Monitor patient's entire body to ensure complete decontamination
B. Transfer patient to clean area
1. Cover floor with plastic sheeting from stretcher to door
2. Patient should be transferred by others not involved in the decon tamination
C. Provide explanations to patient and family to diminish anxiety

EVALUATION

I. Patient outcomes/criteria
A. Complete decontamination as evidenced by clear Geiger counte count
B. Adequate ventilatory status
II. Document initial assessment data, emergency department interventions and patient's response to treatment
III. If previous patient outcomes are not reached, the emergency nurse should reevaluate the interventions and change the plan of care accordingly

DISPOSITION

I. Admission criteria
A. Presence of severe nausea and vomiting
B. Presence of thrombocytopenia, granulocytopenia, and lymphopenia
II. Depends on number of casualties; mass situations will alter indications for care
III. Discharge guidelines
A. Provide instructions for follow-up care for repeat blood counts

SUPPLIES FOR USE IN RADIATION EMERGENCY

Most geographical areas have a designated radioactive substance–control receiving hospital. However, emergency departments should be prepared to handle potential victims from on-site contaminations or isolated contaminations.

Many of the following items are commonly found in emergency departments. If these items are not easily accessible, it is important to know where they can be obtained.

1. Geiger counter
2. Film badges
3. Ring badges
4. Self-reading dosimeters
5. Disposable surgical scrub suits
6. Disposable surgical gowns
7. Plastic shoe covers
8. Surgical caps
9. Surgical masks
10. Surgical gloves
11. Adhesive tape
12. Plastic sheets and bags
13. Plastic sheeting (to be used if the patient walks in the emergency department)
14. Plastic containers for collection of decontamination fluids
15. Radiation "mark-off" rope
16. Assorted radioactive signs and labels
17. Filter papers for smears
18. Spare batteries for radiation detectors
19. Clipboard, paper, and pens
20. Assorted containers for sample collection

A standard medical emergency plan should consist of the following:

1. A list of key personnel (emergency care physician, radiologist, health physicist)
2. A list of emergency supplies
3. A designated medical radiation area or room
4. An established procedure for preparing the radiation room to receive the accident victim
5. Procedures for evaluation of the patient's contamination status
6. Procedures for gowning and protection of hospital personnel
7. Instructions for securing and safely isolating contaminants removed from the patient
8. Procedures for controlling entry into the radiation emergency area
9. Procedures and guidelines for surveying emergency transportation personnel, vehicles, and equipment

CHAPTER 41

SURFACE TRAUMA: WOUND MANAGEMENT

IMPLICATIONS FOR ACTION

This care plan outlines the care required for various types of wounds, bite and stings. Controversies exist concerning specific treatment for these injurie therefore management may vary among emergency departments.

ASSESSMENT

I. Initial observation
   A. Location and appearance of wound
   B. Amount of bleeding
II. Subjective assessment
   A. Source and mechanism of injury
   B. Time of injury and prehospital care
   C. Tetanus immunization status and allergies
III. Objective assessment
   A. Vital signs
   B. Characteristics of wound
      1. Obvious arterial or venous bleeding
      2. Location and depth of wound
      3. Visible underlying structures
      4. Extent of wound contamination or foreign body presence
      5. Local inflammatory response or necrotic tissue
   C. Functional involvement of extremity wound
      1. Vascular: check for five "Ps" of arterial injury (pain, pallor, pulse lessness, paresthesia, and paralysis)
      2. Nerve or tendon involvement: decreased or altered sensation strength, or movement
      3. Bone or joint involvement: decreased movement or increased pain with movement

)SSIBLE NURSING DIAGNOSES/ANALYSIS

.. Comfort, alteration in: pain
[. Fluid volume deficit, actual or potential
[. Knowledge deficit (of wound care)
'. Mobility, impaired physical
'. Skin integrity, impairment of: actual and potential
[. Tissue perfusion, alteration in: peripheral

.ANNING

Priorities for care
A. Control of bleeding
B. Fluid management
C. Cleansing and repair of wound

Differential management (NOTE: Specific cleansing solutions and procedures are outlined in the implementation section)

pe of auma	Clinical Assessment	Management
'OUNDS		
brasions	Damage to epidermis caused by skin rubbing against a hard surface; wound may contain foreign bodies	Scrub to cleanse; may use antibiotic ointment or nonadherent dressing
vulsion	Full thickness skin loss; requires check for tendon, nerve, or muscle injury	Scrub or irrigate or both; may require debridement, suturing
ontusion	Caused by blunt trauma, resulting in extravasation of blood into tissue	Apply ice and give analgesia
aceration	Penetrates through epithelium; requires check for neurovascular, tendon, or muscle damage	May require local anesthetic for exploration; perform irrigation scrub and irrigate for cleansing; wound is usually sutured but depends on etiology
uncture 'ound	Penetration of sharp object through skin; may trap contaminants; requires check for damage to underlying structures	Soak 5-10 minutes in sterile saline and povidone-iodine

Type of Trauma	Clinical Assessment	Management
Foreign Body	May be visual or suspected from etiology of wound	X-ray study recommended to detect glass or metal; depth and size of object determine procedure for removal (NOTE: the nurse should not remove large, protruding foreign bodies; may require surgical intervention)
Traumatic Amputation	Complete amputation of digit or extremity	Digit may be reimplanted if microsurgery is available; place amputated part in container, wrapping it in a sponge soaked with normal saline; surround container with ice; do not expose tissue directly to ice (refer to Chapter 34, Care Plan for Major Multiple Trauma for management of extremity amputation)
BITES AND STINGS		
Human Bites	High incidence of infection, usually cellulitis; often "fight bite" caused when knuckles strike opponent's teeth	Scrub, usually not sutured; administer prophylactic antibiotics
Dog and Cat Bites	Infection most common complication; also occurs with cat scratches	Scrub, usually not sutured; take rabies precautions; administration of prophylactic antibiotics is controversial
Snake Bites		
Nonvenomous	Minimal local swelling or inflammation	Scrub
Venomous	Effects of venom are nausea, vomiting, ecchymosis, local edema, weakness, apprehension, tissue necrosis, hypotension, coagulopathy, neurotoxicity, and hemolysis	Identify snake if possible; measure girth for extremity wound; patient is usually admitted for antibiotics and observation; antivenin available; may require suction and surgical excision

ʻe of ʻuma	Clinical Assessment	Management
ʻder Bites		
ʻlack ʻvidow	Neurotoxin causes muscle cramping, nausea, vomiting, weakness, hypertension	Administer calcium gluconate or methocarbamol (Robaxin) for cramps, analgesics; anti-venin available
ʻrown ʻecluse	Local vasoconstriction, edema, erythema, nausea, vomiting, fever, arthralgia	Nonspecific treatment
ʻes and ʻsps	Localized pain, edema, inflammation, and itching; may cause systemic allergic reaction (refer to Chapter 26, Care Plan for Systemic Allergic Reaction)	Apply ice, elevate, and administer antihistamine
ʻrpions		
ʻNonlethal	Local edema and inflammation	Apply ice, elevate, and administer analgesics
ʻLethal	Systemic findings: hypertension, neurological changes, tachycardia, respiratory difficulty	Provide supportive care

PLEMENTATION

Primary intervention

A. Control bleeding
   1. Apply direct pressure and elevate
   2. Ligation of bleeding vessel by physician; may require formal surgical exploration
   3. Pneumatic tourniquet may be required

B. Manage fluids
   1. Initiate IV of normal saline or lactated Ringer's for presence of
      a) Extensive bleeding or damage
      b) Resting tachycardia
      c) Evidence of concurrent injuries causing hypovolemia
   2. Blood products may be given for extensive hemorrhages

II. Secondary intervention
  A. Obtain laboratory tests
    1. Hematocrit if significant blood loss suspected
    2. Clotting studies for patients with coagulopathy or anticoagula therapy
    3. Type and crossmatch if patient requires transfusion
  B. Obtain x-ray studies to rule out or locate foreign bodies or bony inju
  C. Provide wound management
    1. Specific to physician preference (refer to differential manageme section)
    2. Provide cleansing
      a) Assure sterile conditions
      b) Suture lacerations
        (1) Shave hair 1/4 to 1/2 inch from wound edge; DO NOT SHA EYEBROWS
        (2) Local anesthetic may be required for wound preparation; not use epinephrine on fingers, toes, nose, nipples, or pe because of vasoconstrictive action
      c) Scrub or irrigate wounds with half strength povidone-iodine pr for minimum of 5 minutes; recent trends in some geograph areas are pointing to just using forceful saline irrigation
      d) Do not soak fresh lacerations as edges become too friable f suturing
      e) Rinse wound well with normal saline to remove all povidon iodine solution and cover loosely with sterile dressing
    3. Suturing usually performed by physician
    4. Wounds longer than 8 to 12 hours old usually are not sutured

Schedule for Tetanus Immunization—Adults

No Previous Immunization	Immunized
Tetanus immune globulin 250 units IM Tetanus diphtheria (TD) booster 0.5 ml IM Have patient return for booster shots at 2 months and again 6-12 months later	If last booster >10 years, give tetanus diphtheria (TD) 0.5 ml IM If wound is >24 hours old, neglected, tetanus-prone, give TD 0.5 ml IM if last booster is >1 year

D. Take rabies precautions
   1. Contact local Animal Control to report bites and obtain information of incidence of rabies in area
   2. Describe type, appearance, and behavior of animal
   3. Determine vaccination history of animal if known
   4. Animal will be observed for 10 days
   5. Rabies vaccine is available through State Health agency
E. Administer medications
   1. Provide tetanus immunization for adults and children (refer to tables below)
   2. Administer antibiotics, if indicated, according to physician decision
   3. Administer antivenins
      a) Usually made from horse serum
      b) Give intradermal test before IV dose
F. Offer patient and family explanations of procedures and reassurance

chedule for Tetanus Immunization—Children*

ormal Infants	Children Not Immunized in Early Infancy (15 months-5 years)	Children Not Previously Immunized (5-18 years)†
months: DPT, TOPV months: DPT, TOPV months: DPT, TOPV 2 months: Tuberculin test 5 months: MMR 5-18 months: DPT, TOPV -5 years: DPT, TOPV 4-16 years: TD, repeat every 10 years	First visit: DPT, TOPV, MMR 2 months later: DPT, TOPV Second 2 months later: DPT, TOPV 6-12 months after third visit (or at school entry): DPT, TOPV 14-16 years: TD, repeat every 10 years	First visit: TD, TOPV, MMR 2 months later: TD, TOPV 6-12 months after second visit: TD, TOPV Thereafter: TD, repeat every 10 years

Adapted from the Colorado Department of Health, Colorado Medical Society, Colorado Chap-r of the American Academy of Pediatrics, and the Rocky Mountain Pediatric Society (1/1/80).
There is currently some controversy concerning the value and safety of pertussis vaccine after ;e five. Management should be according to physician preference.

EVALUATION

I. Patient outcomes/criteria
   A. Clean wound
   B. Relief of pain
   C. Approximation of wound edges
II. Document initial assessment data, emergency department interventions and the patient's response to treatment
III. If previous patient outcomes are not reached, the emergency nurse should reevaluate the interventions and change the plan of care accordingly

DISPOSITION

I. Admission criteria
   A. Complicated or multiple injuries
   B. Need for operating room procedure (e.g., tendon repair, debridement) may be handled as outpatient
II. Discharge guidelines
   A. Provide wound care instructions (refer to appendix E)
   B. Give antibiotic instructions
   C. Arrange follow-up visit for wound check or suture removal according to following schedule

Recommended Suture Removal Schedule

Location	Removal in Number of Days
Face	3-5
Scalp	7-10
Abdomen	7-10
Hand	7-10
Arm	7-10
Back	10-14
Leg	10-14

CHAPTER 42

SUTURE REMOVAL

IPLICATIONS FOR ACTION

though usually a simple procedure, it is important to assess for signs of ound infection when a patient comes to the emergency department for sure removal. Extremity or digit motor function should also be checked to sure a return to normalcy. These return visits to the emergency department o offer information related to the patient's compliance with self-care.

SESSMENT

. Initial observation
   - A. Presence or absence of inflammation
   - B. Drainage
   - C. Intact wound edges
   - D. Abnormal swelling

. Subjective assessment
   - A. History of injury
   - B. Care of injury since suturing
   - C. Compliance with home instructional care, such as splinting, antibiotics, or soaks
   - D. Tenderness of wound site

. Objective assessment
   - A. Vital signs, including temperature
   - B. Description of wound
   - C. Gross motor and neurovascular status distal to wound

SSIBLE NURSING DIAGNOSES/ANALYSIS

I. Activity intolerance, potential
I. Knowledge deficit (of care for wounds)
I. Mobility, impaired physical
. Tissue perfusion, alteration in: peripheral
. Self-care deficit: bathing/hygiene
I. Skin integrity, impairment of: actual

PLANNING

I. Follow guidelines for removing sutures (outlined in the table below)

II. If sutures appear imbedded or wound appears very crusted or infecte wound check should be done by physician (refer to Chapter 16, Care Pl for Infection: Localized for discussion of abscess or cellulitis)

IMPLEMENTATION

I. Primary intervention
   A. Clean wound with diluted hydrogen peroxide or normal saline solutio
   B. Clip suture adjacent to skin so least amount of exposed suture materi is pulled through wound

II. Secondary intervention
   A. Cleanse wound with normal saline solution
   B. Apply skin closures to all facial wounds and others as needed
   C. Instruct patient to return if there are any signs of infection, fever, decreased mobility
   D. Provide instructions for wound care, dressing changes, or antibiot therapy if wound is infected

EVALUATION

I. Patient outcomes/criteria
   A. Healing, intact wound with edges approximated
   B. No evidence of drainage or redness
   C. Neurovascular status intact

Recommended Suture Removal Schedule

Location	Removal in Number of Days
Face	3-5
Scalp	7-10
Abdomen	7-10
Hand	7-10
Arm	7-10
Back	10-14
Leg	10-14

I. Document initial assessment data, emergency department interventions, and patient's response to treatment
I. If previous patient outcomes are not reached, the emergency nurse should reevaluate the interventions and change the plan of care accordingly

ISPOSITION

. Send patient home with wound care instructions
. Make follow-up arrangements for wound infection

PART THREE

APPENDIXES

APPENDIX A

PROCEDURES AND PROCEDURE TRAYS

Central Venous Line Placement
Cricothyrotomy
Culdocentesis
Cutdown
Ear, Nose, and Throat Tray
Eye Care Tray
Pacemaker Insertion
Pericardiocentesis
Precipitous Delivery Tray
Peritoneal Lavage
Thoracostomy
Thoracotomy
Uterine Curette Tray

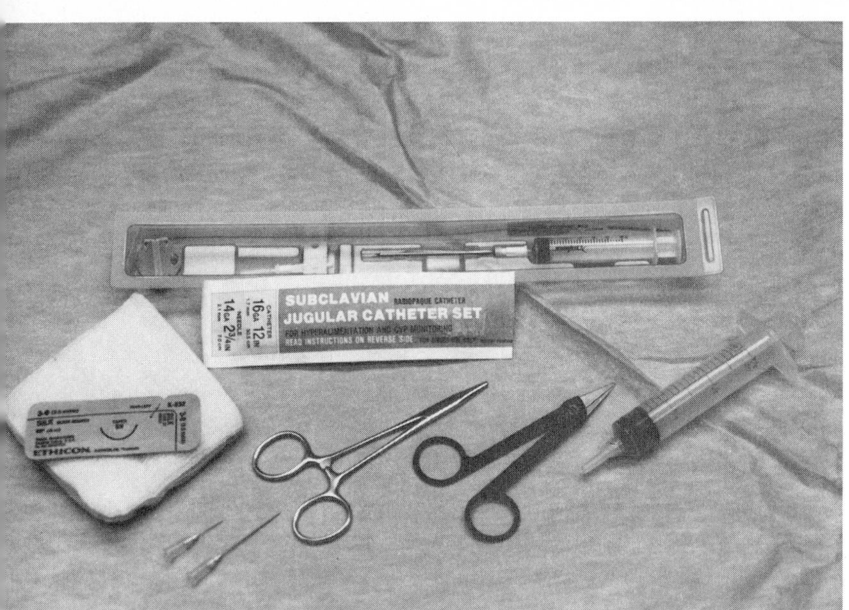

:NTRAL VENOUS LINE PLACEMENT

AY

:eedle holder
uture scissors
4-gauge central venous catheter set
-0 Silk suture package

1 Syringe, 30 ml
1 25-gauge 5/8-inch needle
1 21-gauge 2½-inch needle

DITIONAL SUPPLIES

ocaine 1% for anesthesia
vidone-iodine skin prep
ravenous solution of choice with central venous monitor attached

OCEDURE

Obtain and provide a large central catheter or cordis.

Preflush the intravenous line that has a central venous pressure monitor (CVP) attached with solution of choice.

Provide 3-0 silk suture and needle holder.

The line is usually inserted through the subclavian or internal jugular vein after a povidone-iodine prep.

If chest injuries are present, the insertion site should be on the same side.

Mark the initial reading point on chest wall at the axillary line.

Obtain serial CVP readings to evaluate volume status.

Avoid using the central line for blood transfusions, whenever possible.

Apply an occlusive dressing with povidone-iodine ointment when time permits.

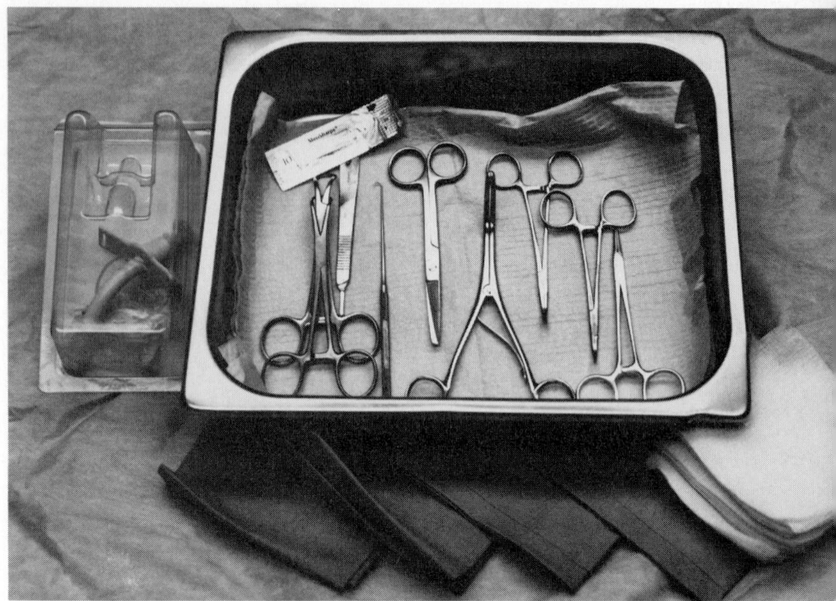

CRICOTHYROTOMY

TRAY

2 Halsted curved mosquito hemostats
1 Webster needle holder, 5 1/2 inch
1 Tracheal dilator
1 Tracheal dilator hook
1 Operating scissors
12 Sponges, 4 × 4 inch
4 Nonabsorbent towels
2 Towel clips
1 Knife handle, #3 blade
1 Knife blade, #11

ADDITIONAL SUPPLIES

1 Syringe, 10 ml
Povidone-iodine skin prep
Lidocaine 1% with epinephrine for anesthesia
Tracheostomy tube, size of choice (in an emergency, a sterile endotracheal tube be used)

PROCEDURE

1. Use the cricothyrotomy tray.
2. Provide a tracheostomy tube; 6.5 mm for average adult.
3. Prep neck with povidone-iodine solution.
4. Prepare suction apparatus and have readily available.
5. Secure the tube after placement with a trach tie or other available tie.
6. Assist with ventilation and suction as needed.
7. Observe for any bleeding at site of procedure.

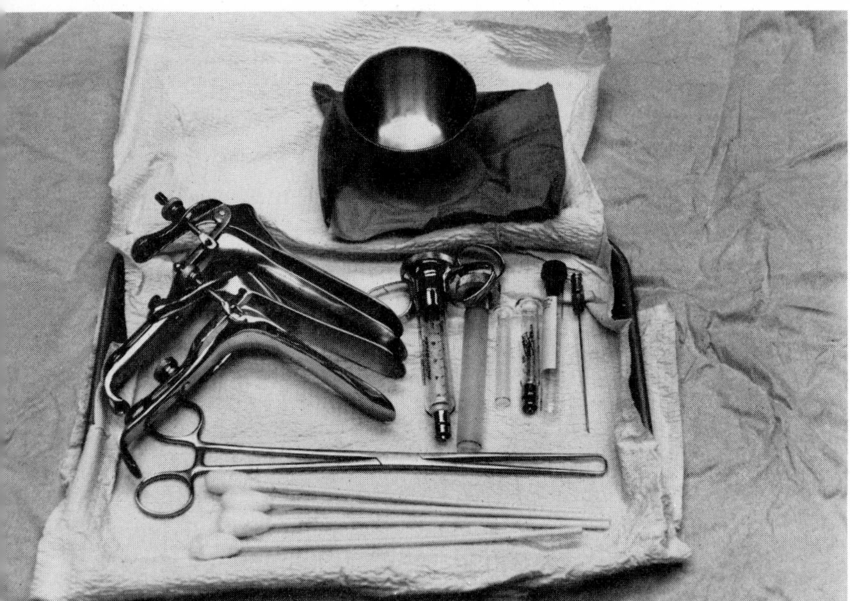

ULDOCENTESIS

AY

Jackson single-tooth tenaculum
Vaginal speculum (medium)
Vaginal speculum (large)
2-inch round basin
Red top laboratory tube

4 Jumbo applicators
1 Syringe ring control, 10 ml
1 Syringe, 2 ml
1 20-gauge $3^1/2$-inch spinal needle
1 21-gauge $1^1/2$-inch needle

DDITIONAL SUPPLIES

esacaine 2% for anesthesia
ovidone-iodine skin prep

ROCEDURE

A diagnostic aid for hemoperitoneum; indicated when ectopic pregnancy is suspected.

Procedure

a) Rectum should be emptied before procedure if possible; enema may be needed.
b) Position patient in lithotomy position; elevate head of bed for pelvic pooling.
c) Have available local anesthetic, spinal needle, and culdocentesis tray.
d) Aspiration from cul-de-sac may show
  (1) A positive tap producing nonclotting blood with a hematocrit >15%; venous or arterial blood should clot.
  (2) A negative tap, which is defined by clear serous fluid; this does not rule out ectopic pregnancy as it may be unruptured.
  (3) A "dry tap," which is nondiagnostic.

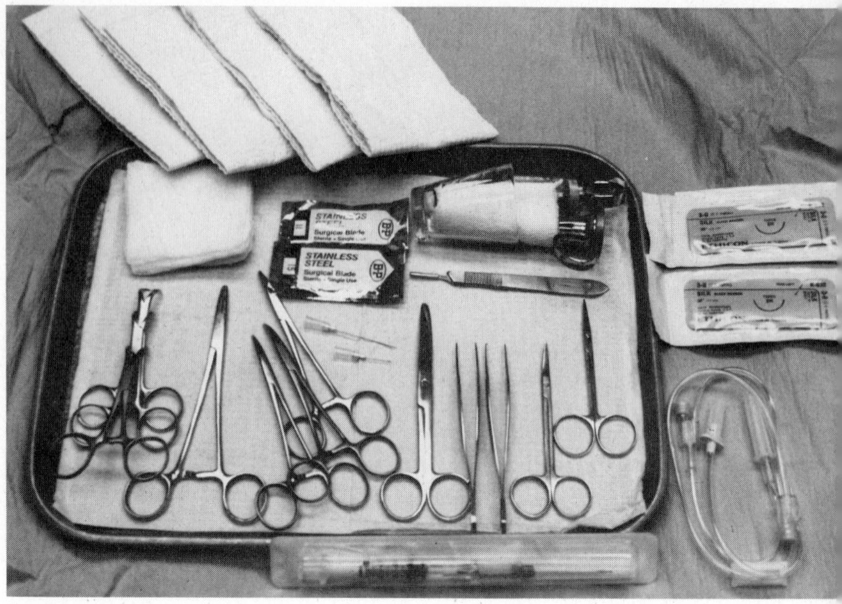

CUTDOWN

TRAY

1 Scalpel handle, #3
1 (each) Knife blades, #11 and #15
1 Iris scissors, curved
1 Iris scissors, straight
1 Adson dressing forceps
1 Adson tissue forceps
3 Halsted mosquito hemostats
1 Webster needle holder
3 Towel clips, 3 inch
1 Suture scissors
1 Syringe, 5 ml, 3 ring
1 25-gauge $5/8$-inch needle
1 21-gauge $1\frac{1}{2}$-inch needle
1 Medicine glass
5 Sponges, 3 × 3 inch
4 Towels, absorbent

ADDITIONAL SUPPLIES

1 14-gauge angiocatheter
1 30-inch extension tubing with two injection sites
Lidocaine 1% for anesthesia
Povidone-iodine skin prep
Intravenous solution of choice with blood administration tubing

PROCEDURE

1. Add large (10–14-gauge) angiocatheter or sterile extension tubing to the cutdo tray.
2. Use a povidone-iodine solution to prep the site.
3. The saphenous vein is most commonly used for insertion.
4. Provide 3-0 silk or 3-0 Vicryl for suturing of the IV in place.
5. Use a blood administration set on IV line; a pressure bag is used when pneum antishock trousers are inflated.

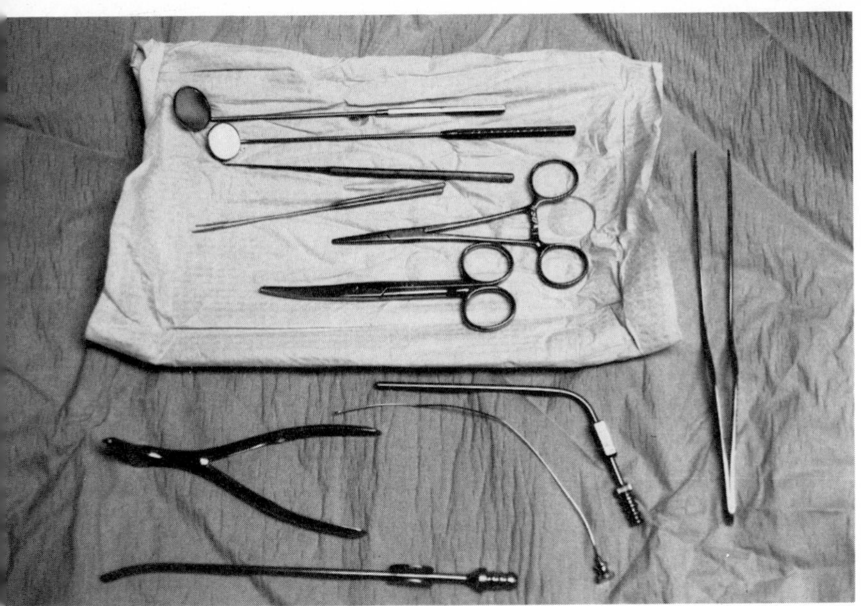

AR, NOSE, AND THROAT

RAY

Operating scissors, sharp, pointed, curved, 5 inch
Crile hemostat, straight, $5^1/_2$ inch
Metal applicators, rough tip
Laryngeal mirrors, sizes 3 and 4
Adson suction tip, 12 fr. with stylet
Cushing bayonet forceps, 7 inch
Vienna nasal speculum

DDITIONAL SUPPLIES

docaine with epinephrine 2% or cocaine 4% or 10% for anesthesia
aseline gauze, 1/4 inch
otton balls
ght source

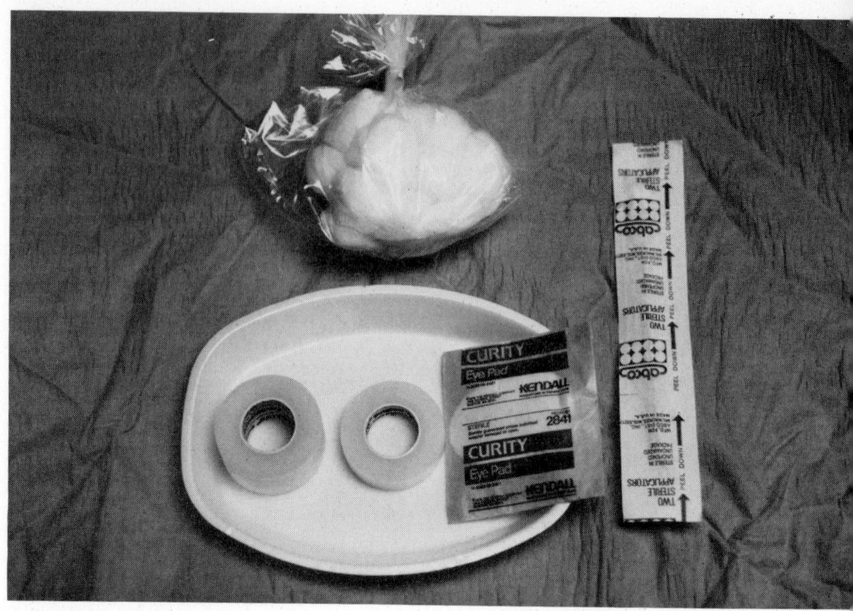

EYE CARE

TRAY

Eye patches
Sterile applicators
Cotton balls
Sterile basin
Tape

ADDITIONAL SUPPLIES

Fluorescein
Sterile irrigating solution
Eye spud
Ophthaine

ACEMAKER INSERTION

ROCEDURE

1. Provide a pacing catheter (size 6 Fr. or 7 Fr.) or transthoracic pacing stylet (with adapter for cables).
2. Provide a pulse generator and cables.
3. Attach limb leads from ECG machine to the patient for monitoring during insertion.
4. Insertion sites that are commonly used
   a) Central site (internal jugular or subclavian) and peripheral site (femoral or brachial) are used in patients with adequate circulatory function (pacer-cath is floated into right ventricle).
   b) Transthoracic site (subxiphoid approach) is used during cardiac arrest or in patients with inadequate circulatory function.
5. All insertion methods require skin preparation with povidone-iodine and aseptic technique.
6. Monitor patient for dysrhythmias during the insertion and have antidysrhythmics and defibrillator readily available.
7. Document capture (QRS complex) per ECG and the threshold (amount of energy needed to produce a QRS).
8. Suture the pacemaker catheter in place with 3-0 silk.
9. Set the pulse generator two to three times above threshold in DEMAND MODE at the desired rate.
10. Secure the pulse generator and cable; it is usually tied to the IV pole.
11. Take a chest x-ray study after insertion to check placement and rule out pneumothorax.

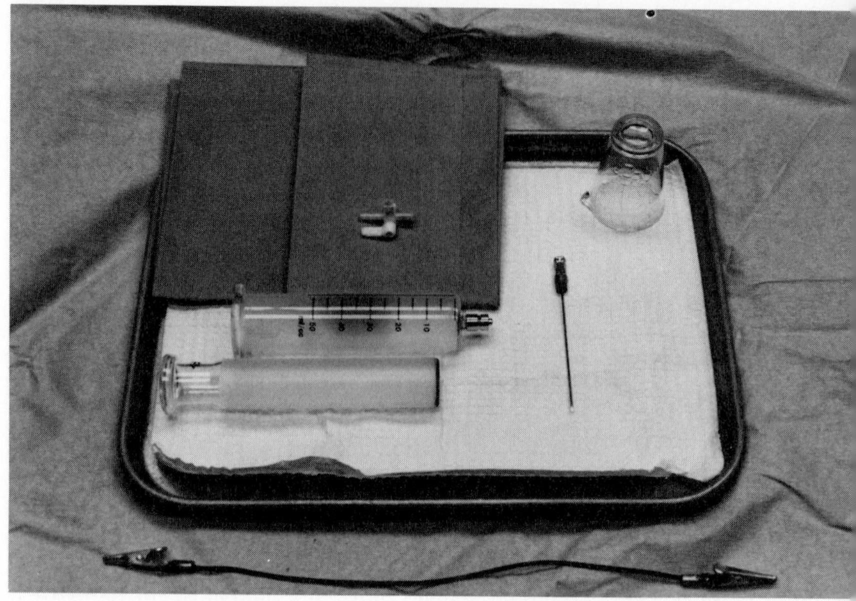

PERICARDIOCENTESIS

TRAY

1 3-way stopcock
1 Medicine glass, 5 ml
1 Glass syringe, 50 ml
2 Nonabsorbent towels
1 18-gauge $3^{1}/_{2}$-inch spinal needle with metal hub

ADDITIONAL SUPPLIES

Alligator clamps
12-lead ECG machine
Povidone-iodine skin prep
Spinal needle, 20 gauge, 3 inch

PROCEDURE

1. Add 20-gauge, 3-inch spinal needle to the tray.
2. Connect an alligator clamp from metal hub to V lead of the ECG machine.
3. Withdraw the spinal needle slightly after noting current of injury resulting fro contact with the myocardium.
4. Withdraw blood and place in glass tube without preservative or anticoagula (commonly a red top tube).
5. Nonclotting blood usually indicates blood from the pericardium.
6. Document the amount of blood withdrawn and the effect on the patient's vital sig tamponade may reoccur, necessitating repeat aspiration.

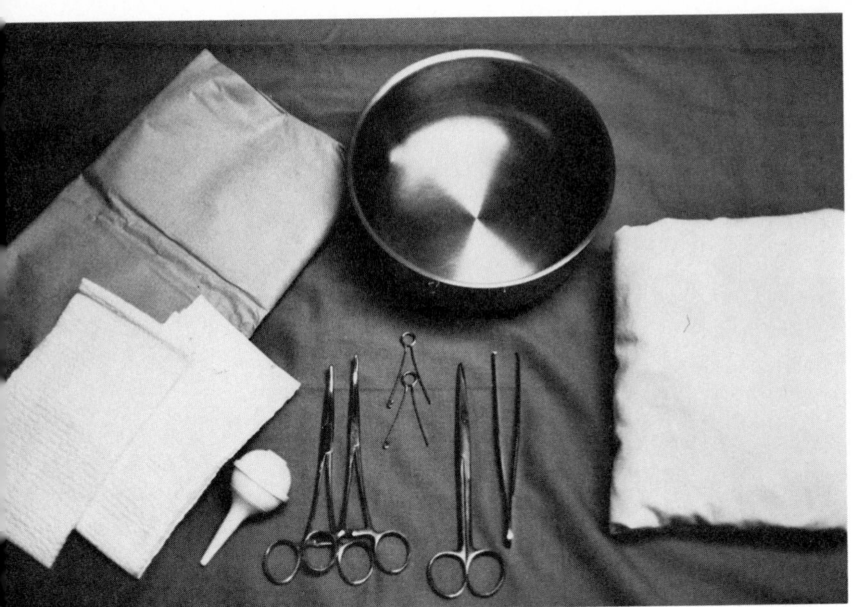

RECIPITOUS DELIVERY

RAY

Drape sheet, 44 × 58 inch
Absorbent towels
Large basin
Mayo scissors, 6 inch
Tissue forceps, 6 inch
Curved Crile hemostats
Clips
Bulb syringe
Baby blanket

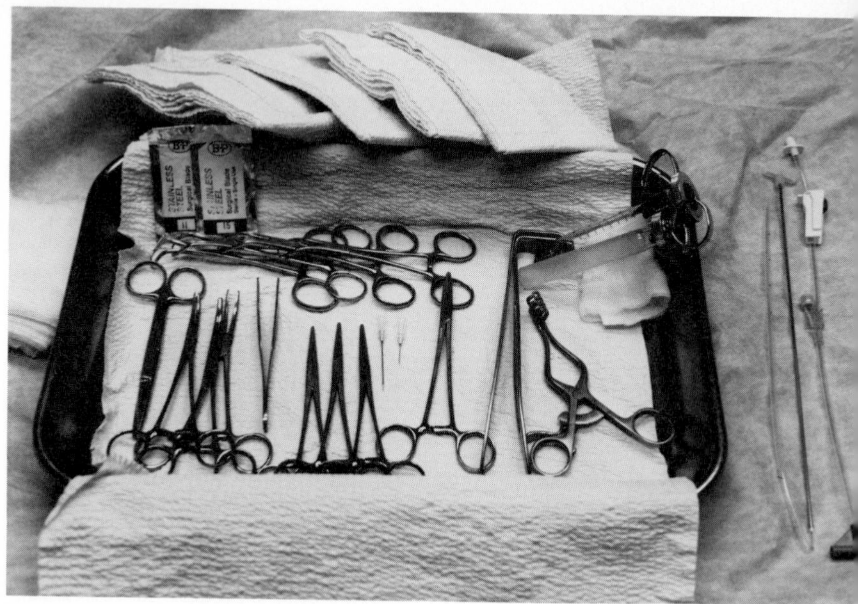

PERITONEAL LAVAGE

TRAY

1 Knife handle, #3 blade
1 (each) Knife blades, #11 and #15
1 Straight suture scissors
1 Tissue forceps, 5 inch
3 Curved Crile hemostats
1 Needle holder, 6 inch
2 Army retractors
1 Weitlaner self-retaining retractor
4 Towel clips
10 Sponges, 4 × 4 inch
1 25-gauge 5/8-inch needle
1 21-gauge 1 1/2-inch needle
4 Nonabsorbent towels
1 Trocath peritoneal dialysis catheter with connecting tubing

ADDITIONAL SUPPLIES

Lidocaine 2% for anesthesia
Razor/prep kit for shaving site
Povidone-iodine skin prep

ERITONEAL LAVAGE

ROCEDURE

Add a peritoneal dialysis catheter and lidocaine to tray.

Before the procedure, insert an indwelling urinary catheter and nasogastric tube.

Shave the infraumbilical area and prep with povidone-iodine solution.

Insert the peritoneal dialysis catheter into the peritoneal cavity.

a) If approximately 10 ml of blood is aspirated, tap is considered grossly positive; patient is taken to the operating room without lavage.

b) If tap is not grossly positive, infuse 1 liter of warm normal saline solution through macro-tubing; for pediatric patients, infuse 15 ml/kg.

c) Let fluid return by gravity by dropping the bag below the patient's bed; do not withdraw fluid for laboratory studies until 750 ml or more has returned.

d) Send the return fluid for cell counts, gram stain, amylase, alkaline phosphate, and bilirubin.

e) Results

   (1) Red cell count of 100,000/ml or more indicates need for surgery.

   (2) Red cell count of 50,000 to 100,000/ml is considered equivocal and treatment is individualized according to clinical status.

   (3) Red cell count of 5000/ml or more with gunshot wounds or concern for diaphragmatic injury indicates need for surgery.

Provide 4-0 prolene and 2-0 polyglectin for closure post-lavage.

Patient is usually admitted to an inpatient unit or kept for 12 hours in an EMS Observation Unit.

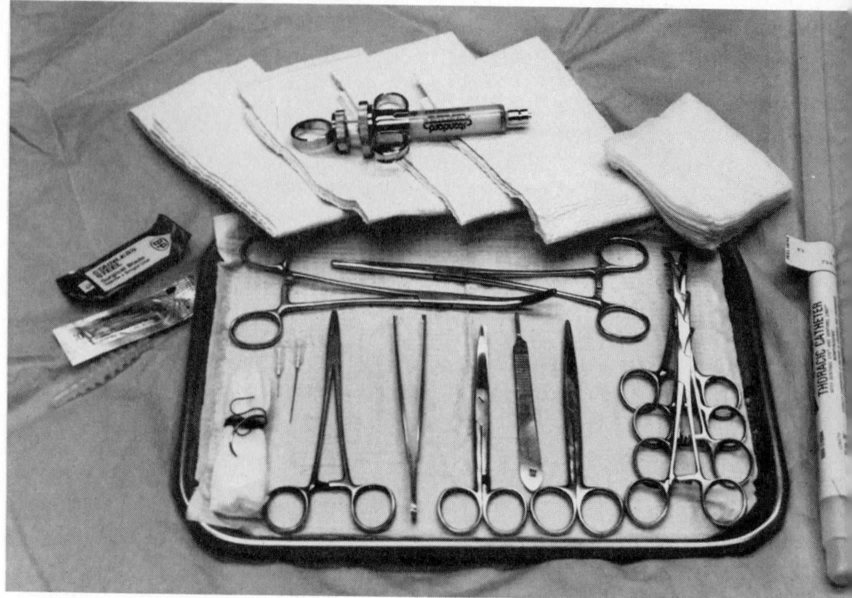

THORACOSTOMY

TRAY

1 Knife handle, #3 blade
1 (each) Knife blades, #10 and #15
1 Scissors, operating, straight
1 Pean forceps, curved, 8 inch or 9 inch
1 Pean forceps, straight, 8 inch or 9 inch
1 Tissue forceps, 5 inch
1 Needle holder, 7 inch
4 Towel clips
1 Mayo scissors, curved, 6 1/4 inch
1 Straight connector, 5 in 1
1 Syringe, 10 ml, 3 ring
1 25-gauge 5/8-inch needle
1 21-gauge 1 1/2-inch needle
6 Sponges, 4 × 4 inch
1 Strand #2 Ethibond suture

ADDITIONAL SUPPLIES

Lidocaine 1% for anesthesia
Povidone-iodine skin prep
Thoracic catheter (chest tube), size of choice (36 to 40 fr. for average adult)
Vaseline gauze
Chest-tube drainage system (style of choice)
Tincture of benzoin
Elastoplast

IORACOSTOMY

ROCEDURE

Add chest tube (36 fr. or 40 fr. for average adult) and lidocaine to tray.

Provide an underwater-seal chest bottle.

Prep the area with povidone-iodine solution.

The chest tube is usually inserted through the fifth intercostal space anterior to midaxillary line into the pleural space.

Connect the chest tube to the chest bottle.

Secure the tube by

a) Suturing at insertion site.

b) Taping the tube connection to avoid a break in the system.

c) Apply an occlusive dressing with vaseline gauze.

Document the amount and type of initial and subsequent drainage.

Note any fluctuation of fluid in tubing.

Maintain the patency of tube by "milking" or "stripping" if clots develop.

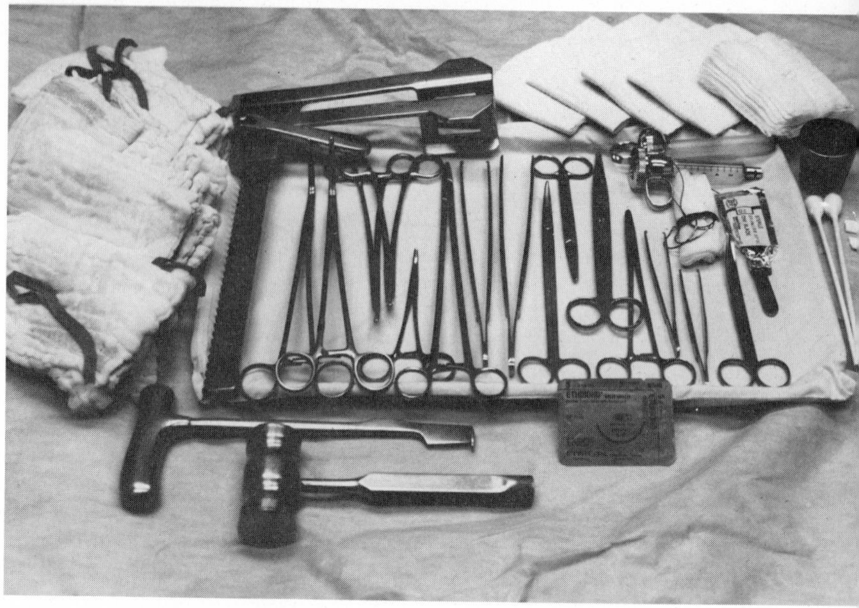

THORACOTOMY

CARDIAC ARREST TRAY

1 Knife handle, #4 blade
1 (each) Knife blades, #10 and #20
1 Mayo scissors, curved, $6\frac{1}{4}$ inch
1 Metzenbaum scissors, 9-10 inch
1 Mayo-Harrington scissors
2 Tissue forceps, $5\frac{1}{2}$ inch
1 Tissue forceps, 10 inch
1 Dressing forceps, 10 inch
2 Pean hemostat, curved, 9 inch
1 Crile hemostat, curved
2 Satinsky vascular clamps
1 Mayo scissors, straight, $6\frac{1}{4}$ inch
1 Metal medicine cup
1 Hegar needle holders, 8 inch and 10 inch
1 Rib spreader
10 lap sponges
1 Syringe, 3 ring, 10 ml
10 Ray-Tec sponges
2 Jumbo applicators
1 Strand, #5 Ethibond suture
2 Teflon pledgets
1 Lepske knife
1 Mallet

DITIONAL SUPPLIES

idone-iodine skin prep

IORACOTOMY (Open Cardiac Arrest Procedure for Internal rdiac Massage)

OCEDURE

Pour povidone-iodine solution over left chest.

A left anterior thoracotomy incision is generally used; if physician decides to transect sternum, a Lepske knife and mallet are required.

Insert rib spreaders; physician then opens pericardium and initiates internal cardiac massage.

Document the time the aortic cross clamp is applied.

Prepare internal defibrillation paddles with sterile saline-soaked gauze if heart is fibrillating; internal defibrillation is usually at 20 to 50 watt/second.

Penetration of myocardium will be temporarily repaired with double-armed cardiovascular suture and teflon pledgets.

Prepare and administer intracardiac or intravenous drugs as ordered by physician.

If cardiac rhythm is reestablished, transport the patient to the operating room for definitive repair.

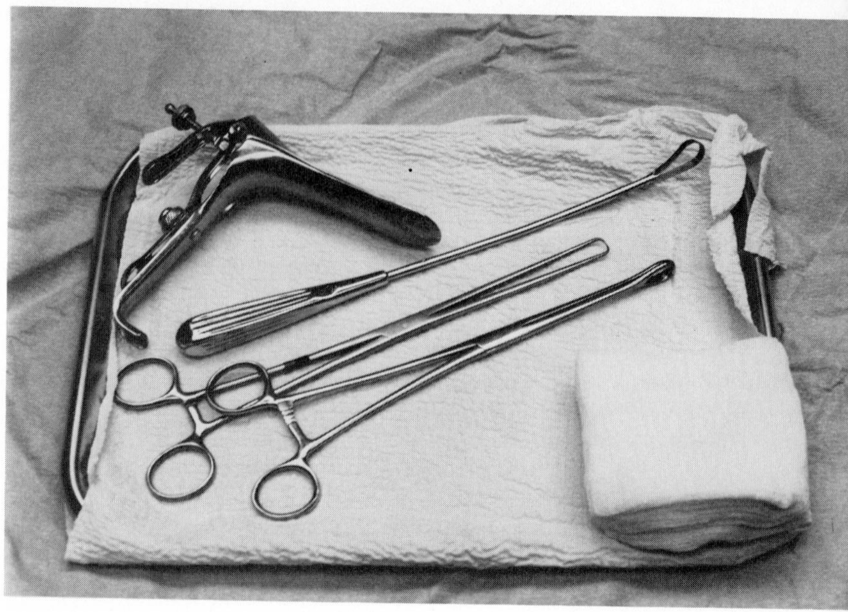

UTERINE CURETTE

TRAY

1 Sims uterine curette, size 4 or 6
1 Jackson single-tooth tenaculum
1 Foerster sponge forceps
1 Medium or large vaginal speculum

ADDITIONAL SUPPLIES

1 Syringe, 10 ml
1 20-gauge $3^1/2$-inch spinal needle
1 21-gauge $1^1/2$-inch spinal needle
Nesacaine 2% for anesthesia
Povidone-iodine skin prep

APPENDIX B

CRISIS INTERVENTION FOR COMMONLY SEEN BEHAVIORAL TYPE PATIENTS

RISIS INTERVENTION

is section will outline crisis intervention considerations for the emergency department, types of difficult behavior problems found in patients, and the mental status amination.

ESCRIPTION OF A CRISIS

General characteristics of all crises

A. Sudden and unexpected
B. The individual, family, or group may not be adequately prepared to handle the event, and normal coping mechanisms are stretched beyond their capacity to produce acceptable behavior
C. Usually short in duration (up to 36 hours)
D. Response to a crisis—whatever the cause of the situation—has the potential to produce dangerous, self-destructive, or socially unacceptable behavior

Fear and anxiety are the basic emotions experienced by all emergency department (ED) patients and may be intensified by

A. Pain
B. Alcohol or other drugs
C. Head injuries
D. Previous emotional or psychiatric problems
E. Unavailability of meaningful, adequate support systems

OALS OF CRISIS INTERVENTION

I. Shield the disturbed person from additional stress
I. Assist the patient and family in organizing and mobilizing available resources
I. Return the patient and family to a precrisis level of functioning

ASSESSMENT

I. Recognizing signs and symptoms of patients who are deteriorating in a crisis situ tion:
   A. Agitation
   B. Hyperactivity
   C. Rapid/slowed speech, which may be characterized by altered vocalization
   D. Gastrointestinal upset
   E. Inactivity
   F. Staring into space
   G. Wandering about aimlessly
   H. Denial of a problem
   I. Mental confusion

II. High priority factors
   A. Is the patient's life or any part of his or her body in danger?
   B. Is there any clear and imminent danger to the caregiver?
   C. Is there need for immediate use of physical/chemical restraints?

III. Secondary factors
   A. What is or seems to be the problem?
   B. Are there others involved in or near the scene of danger?
   C. Consideration that a criminal situation may also exist

INTERVENTION

I. Communication, verbal and nonverbal, is the key tool in crisis assessment afte physical and safety needs have been met

II. It is important to communicate that
   A. The patient will be accepted as a unique individual
   B. Provision will be made for the patient's privacy if this doesn't interfere wit control of dangerous behavior to self or others

III. Common communication blockers to be alert for are
   A. Power, real or imagined
   B. Power identification and its meaning to the patient regarding both himself an the caregiver
   C. Incongruent goals of the caregiver and the patient
   D. Lack of rapport, felt rather than verbally expressed
   E. Attitudes of both patient and caregiver
   F. Prejudices of both patient and caregiver
   G. Differing frames of reference of the patient and caregiver
   H. Language skills
   I. Comfort of the speaker and listener
   J. Environmental distractions

IV. Strategies
   A. General intervention guidelines
      1. No two patients are alike; no caregiver has "seen it all"
      2. All patients have differing expectations of what they want and expect to receive, thus no one "tip" will always work
      3. The interrogatory approach works well in physical medicine but may be only selectively useful in the assessment of emotional, psychological, and behav-ioral problems

4. Violence or behaviorally acting out is a defense, an attempt to maintain control and to release frustration when other resources are unavailable to the patient; it may be stimulated by imprudent physical moves from the medical worker
5. For maximum information, the patient must feel the environment is private, calm, and safe
6. Keep in mind that the patient may have an organic problem that must be treated along with a behavioral problem
7. All persons have civil liberties such as the right to privacy, right to respect as a unique individual, and right to confidentiality; these rights must be considered when providing care
8. Maintain all evidence and report to authorities all incidents mandated by law
9. Keep complete, accurate documentation of all observations, findings, and interventions

B. Safety strategies
   1. DO NOT TAKE ANY UNNECESSARY RISKS!
   2. Do not attempt to disarm a patient without special training
   3. Protect yourself by remaining near exits; do not position yourself in the corner of a room or near equipment that may be used as a weapon
   4. Do not attempt to restrain a patient without an adequate number of trained personnel
   5. Do not attempt to touch the patient until things have calmed down or unless adequate help is available
   6. If restraints are indicated for the protection of the patient and staff, first attempt to use only the magnitude of restraint, chemical or physical, that will most quickly assist the patient to gain self-control

C. Communication strategies
   1. A controlled, calm, nonjudgmental attitude by all caregivers must be imparted to the patient
   2. Be alert to your own and the patient's verbal and nonverbal communications
   3. Listen carefully
   4. Focus on the main problem, then address other problems one at a time
   5. Be truthful; do not promise what you do not know or cannot deliver
   6. Do not argue with the patient
   7. Do not moralize or argue over reality; it is unnecessary to enter the patient's delusional system
   8. Do not take the victim's emotions or behavior personally; it is not necessary to be angry because the patient is angry
   9. Allow the patient to adequately express himself or herself
   10. If possible inform the patient of what you are doing and why
   11. Ask for help if
       a) An impasse occurs
       b) The situation becomes too tense, or you feel you are unable to handle the situation physically, emotionally, or medically
   12. Take your time unless a medical emergency exists or physical danger exists to the patient or staff
   13. Solicit information and help from family and friends when possible

D. Factors common to all interventions
   1. Be practical
   2. Consider immediate needs
   3. Be action/goal-oriented
   4. Make an organized effort
   5. Take actions within the capabilities of the medical personnel and institutio
   6. Make the intervention with the patient's involvement and support when po sible
   7. Continually reassess the situation to make sure the most important needs the patient are being met

TYPES OF DIFFICULT BEHAVIOR PATIENTS*

I. Emotional and psychiatric patients (acute and chronic)
II. Aggressive/assaultive patients
III. Alcohol and substance abuse patients
IV. Suicidal patients
V. Grieving patients and families

DIFFICULT BEHAVIOR PATIENTS

I. EMOTIONAL AND PSYCHIATRIC PATIENTS (ACUTE AND CHRONIC)

Good observational and interpersonal skills are needed in the assessment, interventio and management of a wide range of behaviors and personality traits found in individu als. Determining the degree of disturbance or maladaptive behavior is accomplishe through observation and a mental status examination, the outline of which follows the end of this appendix section.

Inappropriate behavior, appearance, emotional reactions, sensorium, thoug content, or judgment may be the initial indicator that intervention is needed. Con munication with individuals who have disturbances in these areas may be difficult establish and interpret in a limited amount of time. The presence of a severe emotion or thought disorder may not always be characterized by bizarre or uncontrolled be havior, thus the assessment phase of the patient's condition must be amended as add tional data is collected.

Depending on the situation, it may or may not be necessary to ask what th patient's chief complaint or request is. The patient exhibiting emotional extremenes (ranging from extreme apathy or unresponsiveness to wildly euphoric or out-of-contro speech, thought, or behavior) may volunteer a perception of the problem that brough him or her to the medical personnel's attention.

A psychiatric emergency exists when an individual is unable to adapt to and cop with stress, whether external or internal. The intensity, duration, and expression of th stress the individual experiences must be determined.

Transient or situational disorders may occur to any person as a result of sever physical injury, disaster, or an emotional encounter that produces prolonged or over whelming stress. These crisis-producing events are usually short-term and may onl

*A brief description of the assessment of each of these follows.

ially overpower the coping mechanisms of the individual. Usually all that is necesy is recognition and quick intervention, allowing the person to ventilate and explore utions to resolve the problem.

Anxiety and depression, on the other hand, are long-term manifestations of dis-tion of a person's normal function resulting from fear or hopelessness. Normal or timistic assessments of reality are impossible. Episodes of anxiety or depression may quite severe and long lasting, but there are no hallucinations, delusions, or severe, arre thought disorders. These patients come to the emergency department episodi-ly seeking help to control their symptoms (such as suicidal thoughts) and may not vays require inpatient management.

Psychosis represents the most severe form of emotional thought disturbance. This ndition is characterized by long-term severe disruptions of thought and emotional sponses, resulting in an inability to perform activities of daily living. These states are sociated with disorganized thinking, delusions, hallucinations, emotional extremes, d disturbances of motor behavior (e.g., overactivity, pacing, repetition of acts, maintance of fixed posture or gaze).

. AGGRESSIVE/ASSAULTIVE PATIENTS

l patients have the capability to be verbally or physically assaultive depending on ents, feelings, or conflicts that may or may not be controllable. Organically this be-vior may be brought on by a specific cerebral anatomical or metabolical dysfunction. oth psychological and functional causes are usually associated with character or ought disorders.

Assessment through observation, followed by quick intervention, should focus on ow severe the outburst is to the individual and others in his or her environment. The e of physical or chemical restraints should be determined by the setting and the egree and duration of the aggression. The use of any restraints requires more, not less, tention by staff members since such patients may continue to injure themselves. nysically subduing a patient should not be attempted unless there is an adequate num-er of trained personnel to do this since more physical harm may be done to the patient nd staff during a physical altercation than otherwise.

Being alert to escalating anger, frustration, and fear may help medical personnel revent the patient from losing psychological, intellectual, or emotional control and elying on a purely physical defense mechanism.

I. ALCOHOL AND SUBSTANCE ABUSE PATIENTS

ubstance abuse—the deliberate, excessive, and persistent use of any chemical that ters a person's physiological or psychological state—masks, potentiates, or signifi-antly alters the presence of all other types of emergent conditions. Alcohol is the most videly abused substance and its depressant and stimulant properties cause a myriad of ehavior problems.

There are five general classifications of commonly abused substances:

1. Volatile substances (paint, glue, aerosols)
2. Narcotics
3. Depressants
4. Stimulants
5. Hallucinogens

Different substances elicit different behaviors. The type of response is determin not only by the particular substance but also by the following:

1. Physical characteristics of the person (size, weight, metabolism)
2. Emotional situation/environment
3. Tolerance
4. Personality
5. Presence of other substances
6. Underlying thought-ineffective disorder or depressive state

Assessment of individuals suspected of substance abuse requires acute observ tion of signs, symptoms, and behaviors. The patient must be assured that direct que tioning as to the therapeutic, recreational, accidental, or intentional (e.g., suicide tempt) use of all prescribed and self-prescribed substances is necessary only for t patient's physical safety (physical assessment and medical management of substan abuse patients has been discussed in the Care Plans for Chapter 2, Alcohol Intoxicatio Chapter 3, Alcohol Withdrawal; Chapter 20, Poisoning; and Chapter 27, Unresponsi Patient).

The assessment and response of these patients depends on the degree of disru tive and maladaptive behavior exhibited. Behavior may or may not be controllable b the patient because of the effects of the substances abused. Moving the patient to private, calming environment before attempts at interviewing are made is helpful bu not always safe. The patient may not know or truthfully impart to you informatio concerning the substances or amounts ingested. It is important for medical personnel keep in mind that any behaviors may be time-limited; for example, the quiet patient ma suddenly become violent and destructive. Friends and family may be helpful in provic ing information and calming the patient.

IV. SUICIDAL PATIENTS

Recognition and sensitive intervention may be lifesaving for persons contemplatin suicide. Attempted and completed suicides evoke complicated emotional response The incidence of suicide in the general population is high; it is thought that 70% of th population has contemplated suicide at one time, and successful suicide is the tent leading cause of death in the United States. It is estimated that females attempt suicid three times more often than males, but males commit successful suicide three time more often than females.

The lethality and the mode chosen along with an index of recognized risk factor provide significant information. The suicidal patient must be assessed by two simul taneous parameters: the medical seriousness and the psychiatric seriousness of the at tempt. These considerations may not be concordant and it is a common mistake t underestimate the psychiatric seriousness because a medically trivial method was cho sen. The patient may finally succeed if casually dismissed as psychiatrically gesturing o acting out. Conversely, other patients may be in great medical danger despite thei initial, less than deadly intent. Focusing on only one parameter must be avoided.

Listed below are five common patterns of suicide:

1. Suicide of impulse
2. Psychotic depression
3. Suicide to escape suffering
4. Pathological grief response
5. Suicide to communicate thoughts or feelings

The precipitating event may not be known. The goal of emergency management potential suicidal victims is to assess the short-term, immediate risks of suicide. g-term risks are difficult to predict accurately. Listed below are known risk factors ced with lethal outcomes:

1. Individual's present emotional and psychological state
2. Past attempts or diagnosis of psychotic depression
3. Environment and degree of social integration
4. Help resources available to the person (personal, community, financial)
5. Present and past use of alcohol and drugs
6. Previous attempts, onset of destructive behavior
7. Availability and contemplated methods (lethality and publicity of the event, which suggests degree of intent or ambivalence)
8. Precipitating events such as:
   a) Diagnosis or belief one has a major illness
   b) Loss of a loved one
   c) Termination of a close relationship
   d) Economic loss
   e) Change in social status
   f) Failure to achieve personal goals

GRIEVING PATIENTS AND FAMILIES

ere is no way to minimize the impact of death in emergency care. With the continual vancement of technological and mechanical avenues of treatment, medical person-l's role is to relieve suffering, salvage life, and appropriately manage death. As issues ch as the quality of life are explored, the concept of "meaningful death" becomes re the responsibility of caregivers. The attitudes expressed and the manner in which dical personnel treat families and friends dealing with a dying family member or end directly influence the survivors' ability to proceed with a healthy grieving ocess.

It is often in an emergency setting that this process is initiated. Involvement with tragedy of others evokes personal feelings of discomfort, doubt, empathetic identifi-tion (pity, fear), and a sense of failure. The medical personnel's involvement with the nificant others of the deceased patient may be brief, but it has a prolonged impact on the family. When successfully managed, this interaction may provide a unique urce of satisfaction for caregivers.

An understanding of the grief process is necessary for caregivers, but it is the tial notification that death or imminent death is expected that requires sensitive in-vention. A short period of preparation gives the family time to begin to examine the elihood of death and may help to blunt the impact of the eventual news.

After the family has been notified of the death—usually by the doctor—the ergency nurse can best serve by being available to the family, by offering to answer estions, and by explaining further what has occurred.

Providing privacy, without isolation, is optimal. Privacy permits the expression d acceptance of sorrow. The initial response to death is usually expressed as psychic in, an incapacitating 5 to 10 minutes of acute grief. It is important to remain non-dgmental and supportive during the individual's grief reaction, especially as the per-nal and cultural expressions of grief vary and may be totally different from your own.

Viewing of the deceased's body is an option that needs to be presented becau this sight confirms the reality of death for many people. Allowing the family time be together provides them with the opportunity to explore coping strategies a strengthen support systems with each other.

Frequently families need to be given permission to go home, indicating that th have done all that they could and should do. Offering some anticipatory guidance abo the next steps to be taken may help them to move onward from the actual death. T use of sedating medications to blunt the pain of death is discouraged because medic tion only questionably relieves the pain and anxiety and simply prolongs the grievi process.

A follow-up call to the family, should they desire, allows them to ask questions voice concerns that they may still have. This gesture also indicates to the family that t hospital is a caring place and need not be associated only with the death that has ju occurred.

MENTAL STATUS EXAMINATION

The purpose of a mental status examination is to distinguish organic from though affective disorders. The former disorders must be assessed and managed medically, t latter, behaviorally. This distinction aids in the detection and identification of psych pathology and may indicate etiological factors. All aspects of the patient's behavior a data. Components of a mental status examination include evaluating the following:

I. Initial appearance and behavior
   A. Dress
   B. Posture
   C. Facial expressions
   D. Motor activity
   E. Physical characteristics, body configuration
   F. Mood
   G. Reaction to interviewer
   H. Specific mannerisms
II. Speech
   A. Quality of speech
   B. Quantity of speech
   C. Organization of speech
III. Content of thought
   A. Symptomology involving thought (suicidal, obsessive, phobic, paranoid, pow thoughts)
   B. Somatic preoccupations
   C. Symptomology affecting perceptions (delusions, hallucinations)
   D. Other unclassified types of experiences (dreams, déjà vu experiences)

Examination of cognitive functions

A. Orientation
B. Attention, concentration
C. Memory (recent, past)
D. Information and vocabulary, general IQ indicators
E. Abstract reasoning
F. Judgment
G. Perception and coordination (psychomotor)

APPENDIX C

ACUTE OBSERVATION UNIT POLICY*

PURPOSE

To establish guidelines for admission, recordkeeping, and medical and nursing respo sibility for patients admitted to Emergency Medical Services 12-hour Acute Observati Unit.

POLICY

The primary purpose of the Emergency Medical Services Acute Observation Unit is provide care for patients who would benefit from a short-term course of therapy, p tients awaiting a disposition, and patients who require a self-limited period of observ tion.

PRACTICE

The following procedure will be followed when patients are admitted to the Emergen Medical Services 12-hour Acute Observation Unit. There will be a shorter time limit f those patients where it is deemed appropriate. This unit is *not* able to provide critic care/coronary care monitoring.

ADMISSIONS

1. ALL PATIENTS MUST INITIALLY BE EVALUATED IN THE EMERGENCY DEPAR MENT.
2. All admissions must be approved by the emergency department (ED) attending ph sician or senior resident. The admitting note and orders must be countersigned b the ED attending physician or senior resident BEFORE THE PATIENT IS PLACED I THE UNIT.
3. All admissions must be for an anticipated period of greater than 1 hour, but no mo than 12 hours.
4. The capacity of the observation area shall be eight (8) patients.
5. The ED attending physician will take the responsibility for continuous care of th patient. In the case where a consulting service has advised an observation unit a mission, the consulting physician must also take responsibility for monitoring th patient.

*Reprinted with permission of Denver General Hospital, Emergency Medical Services, Denver, Colorado.

All pertinent information concerning changes in a patient's status must be related to the ED attending physician by the ED nurse. Ultimate responsibility for the care of the patient will belong to.the ED attending physician.

All patients with potential surgical problems must have a surgical consultation before admission to the observation unit. Therefore, all surgical patients will be the joint-service responsibility of the observation unit and the Surgery Department.

TIENTS QUALIFYING FOR ADMISSION

Patients for whom a period of observation would yield a diagnosis (8-hour time limit) of

a) Head injury (uncomplicated)

b) Drug overdose, whose management is uncomplicated

c) Undefined abdominal pain

d) Alcohol intoxication where underlying disease has not been excluded

Patients needing short-term therapy who have demonstrated response to earlier therapy for

a) Asthma

b) Dehydration (hydration) requiring more than 2 hours of treatment

c) ED postdilation and curettage or outpatient surgery; such patients must have been treated in the ED; does not include patients recovering from general anesthesia

d) Chronic obstructive pulmonary disease (COPD)

Patients requiring observation while awaiting inpatient beds (2-hour time limit)

a) Patients awaiting transfer to operating room (OR)

b) Patients awaiting transfer to ward bed

c) Patients awaiting transfer to another hospital

Social Service dispositions in which Social Service is either unavailable or is unable to place the patient immediately; this will be permitted only for those patients in this category where extreme need is proven

a) Nonambulatory "overnight guests"

b) Nursing home placement

c) Nighttime discharge

Psychiatric dispositions

a) Mental health transfers

b) Patients needing a short trial of medications

c) Patients awaiting an inpatient psychiatric bed

TIENTS NOT QUALIFYING FOR ADMISSION

Patients requiring fecal disimpaction and enemas.

All patients recovering from sedative/hypnotic medications and general anesthesia purposefully given for elective procedures, unless a complication develops that would necessitate a period of prolonged observation.

Patients requiring critical-care monitoring, which includes respirators.

Patients for whom death is the expected outcome. They will be admitted to an appropriate inpatient service.

The unit will NOT be available for patients receiving elective therapy in clinics such as blood or chemotherapy.

6. No pediatric patients will be admitted. Should a deviation from this rule be need it must be cleared with the ED attending physician, and a mandatory pediatric co sultation must be obtained before admission (daytime clinic resident, evening ministrative resident)
7. Exceptions are transfer patients initially seen in ED and found to be in urgent need blood.

ENTRY INTO THE UNIT

Admission to the unit will be at the order of the ED attending physician in conjuncti with ED charge nurse to assure adequate staffing for both patient numbers and t complexity of cases.

RESPONSIBLE PERSONS

One full-time RN
ED attending physician: responsible for each patient
Hospital attendant
When appropriate, a joint inpatient-service consulting physician
Responsibilities: Attending physician and RN write a progress note on each patie including specific physician orders. Progress note by the attending physician a RN will be required every 8 hours. In addition, the physician from the consulti service must also write a progress note. A physician discharge note and order m be written before any patient can leave the unit.

EXTENDED STAY

There should be no extended stays beyond 12 hours. Patient status must be evaluat to assess potential for inpatient admission or discharge home or to another facility.

DISCHARGES

1. Home
2. An inpatient unit
3. Another facility

GENERAL COMMENTS

1. All attempts should be made to have IVs started, NG tubes inserted before admissio
2. No one will be directly triaged to the observation unit. All patients must be eval ated in the ED or outpatient clinic before admission.
3. The nurse assigned to the unit is responsible for monitoring compliance with 8-ho progress notes and proper admission and discharge orders. The ED attending phys cian or the senior resident should be reminded before shift change at 0700, 150 and 2300 hours of any incomplete records on Acute Observation Unit patients.

APPENDIX D

GUIDELINES FOR OBTAINING ORGANS FOR DONATION

y individual who enters the emergency department without prior significant medical story and is presumed brain dead should be considered as a potential organ donor. ere is a critical need for donors; therefore it is the emergency nurse's role to help the ysician identify donors, notify the nearest transplant center, obtain consent, and aintain the donor's vital functions. Organ donations are needed for eyes, kidneys, ear nes and eardrums, pituitary glands, skin, livers, hearts, and bones. Guidelines for the anagement of the event are:

. Identify the donor
   - A. Arrival in emergency department
     1. Unconscious
     2. Heartbeat intact
     3. Respirations intact or assisted
     4. Adequate urine output
     5. Fixed and dilated pupils and no reflexes
     6. Death pronounced for clear medical reasons and never by members of transplant team
   - B. Chief complaint
     1. Acute head injury
     2. Cerebral vascular accident
     3. Drug overdose
     4. Smoke inhalation
   - C. Age: newborn to 60 years
   - D. Past medical history
     1. No sepsis or active communicable diseases
     2. No malignancies
     3. No malignant hypertension
     4. No renal disease
     5. No real or suspected homicide
   - E. Laboratory tests
     1. BUN
     2. Creatinine

3. Liver function test
4. Hepatitis antigen
5. Syphilis screening
6. Blood typing
7. Urinalysis, culture and sensitivity
8. 70 ml of heparinized blood for transplant team

II. Notify transplant center
  A. Notify center of potential donor
  B. Representative may help in obtaining consent

III. Obtain consent
  A. Uniform Anatomical Gift Card
    1. Must have two witnesses
    2. Drivers license is legal for consent in some states but not all
  B. Next of kin
    1. Always get permission from next of kin—even if donor card is with patie
    2. Ask for multiple organs

IV. Maintain vital functions
  A. Blood pressure
    1. Maintain systolic pressure between 140 to 70
    2. Dopamine: drug of choice for hypotension
    3. Use crystalloids to maintain volume and perfusion of organs
    4. Corneas can be transplanted without maintenance of perfusion (see belo
  B. Urine output
    1. Should be maintained at 50 ml/hr or above
    2. Other organs can be used even if kidneys are not viable
  C. Temperature
    1. Maintain at >95 degrees F
  D. Respirations on ventilator

The patient should be transferred from the emergency department to an intens care unit where brain death will be confirmed. The coroner usually must give perm sion in certain cases of the following: head trauma, overdoses, smoke inhalation, when legal problems are a contributing factor.

Treatment of patient after pronouncement of brain death for eye donation.

1. Ensure eyes are moist. Normal saline or artificial tears should be instille eyes are dry.
2. Tape eyes shut carefully. Run tape from forehead to cheek over closed li Wrap small amount of ice (2 tablespoons) in washcloth and place over ey
3. Eyes must be removed within 4 hours of death for viability of the cornea
4. Patients not suitable for eye donation: those with eye trauma. Even disea eyes are useful for research.

APPENDIX E

PATIENT DISCHARGE INSTRUCTIONS (ENGLISH AND SPANISH)*

ıe purpose of providing discharge instructions to patients seen in the emergency ·partment is to clarify and ensure a thorough understanding of the aftercare for the ıtient's presenting problem. The nurse, in conjunction with the primary care physi-an, will provide, on discharge of the patient from the department, the appropriate scharge instruction sheet.

The following guidelines should be followed in issuing instruction sheets:

1. It is the responsibility of the primary care nurse to make sure that appropriate patients receive discharge instruction sheets.
2. If the patient is discharged by the physician without further contact with the nurse, the physician will give the discharge instructions.
3. Documentation is done by the person discharging the patient.
4. Written documentation of which sheets were given to the patients and the initials of who gave the instructions must be placed in the lower left corner of the emergency department chart.
5. The nursing flow sheet has a discharge instruction box that should be filled out and initialed when a flow sheet is used on a patient.

'he following discharge instruction sheets are reprinted with the permission of Denver ·neral Hospital Emergency Medical Services.

ABDOMINAL PAIN

GENERAL INFORMATION

We have done all the tests and examinations that we feel are needed to evaluate yo symptoms. At present, we believe that your abdominal pain will lessen over the next hours. However, we ask that you observe yourself closely and use care in eating.

You may go home at this time if you follow the instructions below:

INSTRUCTIONS

1. Do not eat any solid food for 12 to 24 hours. Drink only liquids like bouillon a gelatin.
2. Take only medicines prescribed by your doctor.
3. Take your temperature in the morning and at night.

CALL OR RETURN TO THE EMERGENCY DEPARTMENT

1. If your pain gets worse or does not go away in 2 days.
2. If your fever increases over 101 degrees F or 38 degrees C.
3. If you become sicker or vomit more frequently.
4. If your pain localizes to one particular area.
5. If you have blood in urine or stool.

RE: ABDOMINAL PAIN

)LOR ABDOMINAL

FORMACION GENERAL

mos hecho todas las pruebas y exámenes que pensamos se indican para evaluar sus tomas. Ahora, creemos que su dolor abdominal va a disminuir en las próximas 24 ras. Sin embargo, pedimos que se observe atentamente y tenga cuidado en lo que ma.

Usted puede ir a su casa si sigue las siguientes instrucciones:

STRUCCIONES

No coma ninguna comida sólida por 12 a 24 horas. Beba solo líquidos como caldo y gelatina.

Tome sólo las medicinas recetadas por su doctor.

Tómese la temperatura por la mañana y por la noche.

AME POR TELEFONO O REGRESE A LA SALA DE EMERGENCIA SI LE PASA SIGUIENTE

Si su dolor se empeora o si no se quita en 2 días.

Si su fiebre aumenta sobre 101 grados F o 38 grados C.

Si se enferma más o si vomita más seguido.

Si su dolor se localiza en un área en particular.

Si tiene sangre en la orina o en el excremento.

---

nslated from English to Spanish by Pauline Manzanares, Denver General Hospital Spanish erpreter.

BURNS

GENERAL INFORMATION

You have a:

☐ First-degree burn, which is a minor burn. It is like a sunburn with redness and pa

☐ Second-degree burn, which is a deeper burn. It has redness and blisters.

☐ Third-degree burn, which is very deep and damages all layers of the skin.

Your skin is a natural barrier to infection. Because the burn has damaged your skin, y must follow these instructions to prevent infection:

INSTRUCTIONS

1. If your burn does not have a dressing on it, you may wash it gently with mild s and water.
2. If your burn does have a dressing on it, follow your physician's instructions:
   ____
   ____
3. If your burn is on an arm or leg, elevate the affected limb as much as possible. T will help keep swelling down and help decrease your pain.
4. Follow-up care:
   ☐ Return to the emergency department to have your burn checked on this d ____________ at ________ AM PM with Dr. ____________
   ☐ Call for an appointment in the surgery clinic in ________ days.
5. Take the following medications as ordered by your doctor:
   ☐ Antibiotic ____________ take ________ times a day.
   ☐ Pain medicine ____________ take ________ pill every ________ hours as needed for pain.

CALL OR RETURN TO THE EMERGENCY DEPARTMENT

1. If there is increased redness, tenderness, or swelling around the burn.
2. If there is pus around or coming from the burn.
3. If you have a fever.

RE: BURNS

UEMADURAS

FORMACION GENERAL

ted tiene:

Una quemadura de primer grado que es una quemadura secundaria. Es como una quemadura del sol, su piel está roja y tiene dolor.

Una quemadura de segundo grado que es una quemadura profunda. Su piel está roja y tiene ampollas.

Una quemadura de tercer grado que es una quemadura muy profunda y daña todas las capas de la piel.

piel es una barrerra natural contra la infección. Porque la quemadura ha dañado su el, usted debe seguir estas instrucciones para prevenir infección:

STRUCCIONES

Si su quemadura no tiene un vendaje puesto, se la puede lavar lentamente con jabón suave y agua.

Si su quemadura tiene un vendaje puesto, siga las instrucciones de su doctor:

____

____

Si su quemadura está en una pierna o en un brazo, levante ese miembro tanto como sea posible. Esto ayudará a mantener la hinchazón baja y ayudará a disminuir su dolor.

Tratamiento complementario de cuidado:

☐ Regrese a la Sala de Emergencia para que revisen su quemadura en la fecha ______________ a las ________ AM PM con el Doctor ______________.

☐ Llame por teléfono para hacer una cita en la Clínica de Cirugía en ________ días.

Tome las siguientes medicinas como ha prescrito su doctor:

☐ Antibiótico ______________________ tome ________ veces al día.

☐ Medicina para el dolor ______________________ tome ________ pastilla cada ________ horas como se necesita para el dolor.

AME POR TELEFONO O REGRESE A LA SALA DE EMERGENCIA SI LE PASA SIGUIENTE

Si está más roja su piel, si aumenta el dolor o si tiene hinchazón alrededor de la quemadura.

Si tiene pus alrededor de la quemadura o si le sale pus de la quemadura.

Si tiene fiebre.

nslated from English to Spanish by Pauline Manzanares, Denver General Hospital Spanish erpreter.

CAST CARE

GENERAL INFORMATION

You have had a cast put on. There are some things you need to do to keep your c clean and comfortable:

INSTRUCTIONS

The cast becomes firm to the touch 10 to 15 minutes after it is applied, but during first 24 hours it is soft and can be easily dented or cracked. After the cast is dry, it m be kept dry or it will crack and crumble.

- An arm or leg cast can be protected during bathing with a plastic bag. Do not lov the cast into water. It may be easier to take a sponge bath while the cast is on.
- If the cast becomes soiled, it can be cleaned with a damp washcloth and a cleanse the area you cleaned is large, expose it to the air or sunlight to dry the plaster. Do put clothing over the cast until it dries.
- The hose of a hair dryer may be used to blow cool air into the cast (set temperatur the hair dryer on "cool"). This may also be used to relieve itching or to dry the c
- If a "walking" cast is applied, do not walk on it for the first 24 hours.

Skin Care:

- Check your skin every day. Press the skin back around all cast edges and look and for reddened areas or sores.
- A reddened area should be rubbed with a small amount of alcohol or lotion.
- DO NOT stick any object under the cast. This may injure the skin.

Follow-up Care:

☐ Return to the emergency department on this date ________________ for y 24-hour cast check.

☐ Call to make an appointment in the orthopedic clinic in ________ weeks.

Take the following medications as ordered by your doctor:

☐ Pain medicine ____________________ take ________ pill every ______ hours as needed for pain.

CALL OR RETURN TO THE EMERGENCY DEPARTMENT

1. If you have tingling or numbness in your toes or fingers.
2. If your toes or fingers are cold to the touch or appear blue.
3. If you have increased pain.
4. If there is a foul smell from the cast or if staining occurs that was not present wh you left the emergency department.

RE: CAST CARE

UIDADO DEL YESO

NFORMACION GENERAL

: han puesto un yeso. Hay algunas cosas que necesita hacer para mantener su yeso npio y cómodo:

NSTRUCCIONES

l yeso se hace duro en 10 a 15 minutos después de que se lo ponen, pero durante las rimeras 24 horas está blando y se abolla y se raja fácilmente. Después que se seca el :so, debe mantenerse seco o se va a rajar y desmenuzar.

Un yeso para el brazo o pierna se puede proteger con una bolsa de plástico cuando usted se baña. No ponga el yeso adentro del agua. Sería más fácil darse un baño con una esponja mientras tiene el yeso puesto.

Si se ensucia el yeso, lo puede lavar con una toalla húmeda y un limpiador. Si el área del yeso que usted limpie es grande, póngalo en el aire o en la luz del sol para que se seque. No ponga ropa sobre el yeso hasta que se seque.

La manguera de una secadora de pelo se puede usar para soplar aire frío en el yeso (ponga la temperatura de la secadora en "frío"). Esto también ayudará a aliviar la picazón o para secar el yeso.

Si le ponen un yeso de "caminar", no camine en él por las primeras 24 horas.

uidado de la piel:

Revise su piel cada día. Apriete la piel hacia atrás alrededor de las orillas del yeso y busque y sienta por áreas rojas o por granos.

Un área rojo debe ser frotado con un poco de alcohol o loción.

NO ponga ninguna cosa debajo del yeso. Eso puede dañar la piel.

atamiento complementario de cuidado:

] Regrese a la Sala de Emergencia en la fecha ______________ para su chequeo de 24 horas de tener el yeso puesto.

] Llame por teléfono para hacer una cita en la Clínica Ortopédica (Orthopedic Clinic) en ________ semanas.

ome las siguientes medicinas como ha prescrito su doctor:

] Medicina para el dolor ______________________ tome ________ pastilla cada ________ horas como se necesita para el dolor.

LAME POR TELEFONO O REGRESE A LA SALA DE EMERGENCIA SI LE PASA O SIGUIENTE

1. Si tiene hormigueo o entumecimiento en sus dedos de los pies o de las manos.
2. Si sus dedos de los pies o de las manos están fríos o se ponen de color azul.
3. Si el dolor le aumenta.
4. Si tiene mal olor del yeso o si tiene manchas el yeso que no tenía cuando se despidió de la Sala de Emergencia.

---

ranslated from English to Spanish by Pauline Manzanares, Denver General Hospital Spanish nterpreter.

COMMON COLD AND FLU

GENERAL INFORMATION

Most colds and the flu are caused by viruses. Viruses cannot be killed by antibioti therefore, they must be killed by the body's own defenses. Cough, headache, sc throat, general body aches, and a runny nose are frequently seen with a cold. Th symptoms usually last 1 week and begin gradually.

Flu symptoms usually start suddenly with a headache and general body aches congested nose and a dry cough may be present. Fevers are usually between 101 to 1 degrees F. These symptoms may last from 7 to 10 days.

INSTRUCTIONS

Although there is no cure for a cold or the flu, the following suggestions may relie some of the symptoms:

- *Fever, aches, and pains:* take aspirin* or Tylenol as directed.
- *Runny nose:* a decongestant may be recommended; increase fluid intake.
- *Cough:* use a humidifier, increase fluids; a cough syrup may be ordered.
- *Sore throat:* gargle with warm salt water every 3 to 4 hours; use throat lozenges.

CALL OR RETURN TO THE EMERGENCY DEPARTMENT

1. If your fever remains higher than 101 degrees F or 38 degrees C for longer than hours while taking aspirin or Tylenol.
2. If you have a severe sore throat.
3. If you have increased coughing or a cough that produces yellow, green, or bloo tinged sputum.
4. If you have sharp chest pain, especially when breathing deeply.
5. If you have pain or discharge from ears.
6. If you have severe pain in the face (sinus) or pain with green or yellow dischar from nose.
7. If you have severe stiffness.

*Note: Aspirin should NOT be given to children.

RE: COMMON COLD AND FLU

L CATARRO COMUN Y LA GRIPE

NFORMACION GENERAL

asi todos los resfríos y la gripe son causados por un virus. Virus no se pueden matar on antibióticos. Por lo tanto, deben ser matados por las defensas de su propio cuerpo. os, dolor de cabeza, dolor de garganta, dolores generales del cuerpo son síntomas que on frecuentemente asociadas con un resfrío. Los síntomas usualmente duran por 1 emana y empiezan gradualmente.

Síntomas de la gripe usualmente empiezan de repente con dolor de cabeza y olores generales del cuerpo. Puede tener congestión de la nariz y una tos seca. Fiebres sualmente suben de 101 grados a 104 grados F. Estos síntomas pueden durar de 7 a 10 ías.

NSTRUCCIONES

unque no hay remedio para un resfrío o la gripe, las siguientes sugestiones pueden liviar algunos de los síntomas:

Para fiebre y dolores, tome aspirina* o Tylenol como le han dirigido.

Para catarro, se recomienda que use una descongestionante. Aumente la cantidad de líquidos que tome.

Para tos, use un humedecedor, aumente los líquidos; un jarabe para la tos se puede usar.

Para dolor de garganta, haga gárgaras con agua tibia con sal cada 3 a 4 horas; use tabletas para la garganta que se chupan.

LAME POR TELEFONO O REGRESE A LA SALA DE EMERGENCIA SI LE PASA O SIGUIENTE

1. Si tiene fiebre más alta que 101 grados F o 38 grados C por más tiempo que 36 horas mientras esté tomando aspirina o Tylenol y no se quita la fiebre.
2. Si tiene dolor muy fuerte de la garganta.
3. Si tiene aumento de tos o una tos que produce saliva de color amarillo o verde o con sangre.
4. Si tiene dolor agudo del pecho cuando respira profundamente.
5. Si tiene dolor o desecho de los oídos.
6. Si tiene dolor fuerte en la cara (senos), dolor con desecho verde o amarillo de la nariz.
7. Tiesura grave.

*Nota: NO se debe dar la aspirina a los niños.

Translated from English to Spanish by Pauline Manzanares, Denver General Hospital Spanish nterpreter.

CRUTCHES

GENERAL INFORMATION

You have been given crutches so you will not use your injured leg while it is healing. you are to put NO weight on your injured leg, your leg is called "nonweight bearing." you can put some weight on your injured leg, your leg is called "partial weight bearin During the beginning period of your recovery, your leg should be nonweight bearing

INSTRUCTIONS

The following instructions will help you with crutch walking:

- Hold your head up and keep your back straight. This will help you keep your balanc
- Put the weight of your entire body on the handgrips with your hands. NEVER PU ANY PRESSURE ON YOUR ARMPITS when walking or standing.

Follow these steps when walking with your crutches:

- Place each crutch tip 4 to 6 inches to the front and side of each foot.
- Move both crutch tips forward on each side 12 to 15 inches from the tip of yo injured leg, while simultaneously moving your injured leg forward 12 to 15 inche
- Then move your uninjured leg forward to the level of the crutch tips.

When going up stairs:

- Keep a crutch under each arm to support your weight.
- Lift your uninjured leg onto the step above with a hopping movement.
- Support your weight on your uninjured leg. Lift both crutches and your injured le onto the step.

When going down stairs:

- Keep a crutch under each arm.
- Place each crutch on the step below. At the same time, swing your injured leg o over the step.
- With your weight on the crutches, step down onto the step with your uninjured leg

CALL OR RETURN TO THE EMERGENCY DEPARTMENT

1. If there is numbness, tingling, or swelling in your arms.
2. If you think your crutches are adjusted wrong (the top of the crutches should be inches or 2 finger-breadths from your armpits).

RE: CRUTCHES

ULETAS

FORMACION GENERAL

han dado muletas para usar para que no use su pierna herida mientras está cicatri-ndo. Si no tiene que poner peso en su pierna herida, eso se dice "soporte sin peso." puede poner peso en su pierna herida, eso se dice "soporte sin peso parcial." Durante período inicial de su recuperación, usted debe poner "soporte sin peso."

STRUCCIONES

s siguientes instrucciones le ayudarán a aprender como caminar con muletas:

Mantenga su cabeza levantada y mantenga su espalda derecha. Esto le ayudará a mantener su equilibrio.

Ponga el peso de todo su cuerpo sobre las agarraderas de las muletas con sus manos.

NUNCA PONGA PRESION DEBAJO DE SUS BRAZOS cuando esté caminando o esté parado.

ga estas instrucciones cuando camine con las muletas:

Ponga la punta de cada muleta cuatro a seis pulgadas hacia adelante y hacia al lado de cada pie.

Mueva las puntas de las muletas hacia adelante 12 a 15 pulgadas, manteniendo las puntas de las muletas a los lados de sus piernas, y al mismo tiempo moviendo su pierna herida hacia adelante 12 a 15 pulgadas.

Entonces mueva su pierna sana hacia adelante hasta el nivel de las puntas de ambas muletas.

ıando suba escalones:

Mantenga una muleta debajo de cada brazo para soportar el peso.

Levante su pierna sana y póngala en el escalón de arriba. Este movimiento es un brinco.

Ponga todo su peso en la pierna sana. Levante ambas muletas y su pierna herida al escalón.

uando baja escalones:

Mantenga una muleta debajo de cada brazo.

Ponga ambas muletas en el escalón de abajo. Al mismo tiempo balancee su pierna herida hacia un lado sobre el escalón.

Con su peso sobre las muletas, baje el escalón con su pierna sana.

LAME POR TELEFONO O REGRESE A LA SALA DE EMERGENCIA SI LE PASA O SIGUIENTE

Si hay entumecimiento o hormigueo en sus brazos.

Si usted piensa que sus muletas están ajustadas mal (la parte de arriba de sus muletas debe estar dos dedos de ancho debajo de sus brazos).

---

anslated from English to Spanish by Pauline Manzanares, Denver General Hospital Spanish terpreter.

DILATION AND CURETTAGE (D & C)

GENERAL INFORMATION

You have had a dilation and curettage (D & C) in the emergency department after y miscarriage. During the D & C, your uterus was cleaned of the remaining tissue f your pregnancy. You will have moderate vaginal bleeding for 4 to 6 weeks. This ble ing will gradually decrease. You will also have mild to moderate lower stomach cra ing.

INSTRUCTIONS

You must follow these instructions after you leave the emergency department:

- Do not put anything into your vagina for 2 weeks. You may not have intercou douche, or use tampons.
- Do not do any heavy lifting for 2 weeks; rest more than usual.

Medications:

These prescriptions were given for medicine to take at home:

- ☐ Methergine 0.2 mg to take every 4 hours. This medication will help your ute return to normal size.
- ☐ Vibramycin 250 mg to take twice a day. This medication is an antibiotic to prev infection.
- ☐ Tylenol with codeine for pain. You may take one or two tablets every 4 hours wh you need it.
- ☐ ______________________________
  ____
- ☐ Call to make an appointment in the GYN clinic in ________ weeks.
- ☐ See your own doctor or go to a health clinic in ________ weeks.

CALL OR RETURN TO THE EMERGENCY DEPARTMENT

1. If your bleeding increases or turns bright red.
2. If you pass large blood clots or tissue from your vagina.
3. If you have a fever over 100 degrees F or 38 degrees C.
4. If you have increasing pain or cramps.
5. If you have a foul-smelling vaginal discharge.

RE: DILATION AND CURETTAGE (D & C)

ILATACION Y LIMPIEZA DE LA MATRIZ

FORMACION GENERAL

sted ha tenido una dilatación y limpieza de la matriz después de su aborto espontáneo. urante éste procedimiento, le limpiaron su utero y le quitaron los tejidos que queda- n adentro durante su embarazo. Va a sangrar poco de la vagina por 4 a 6 semanas. Esto a disminuir gradualmente. También va a tener pocos o moderados cólicos del estó- ago.

ISTRUCCIONES

ebe seguir estas instrucciones después de despedirse de la Sala de Emergencia:

No introduzca nada adentro de su vagina por 2 semanas. No tenga relaciones sexuales, no se duche, y no use tampones.

No levante nada pesado por 2 semanas; descanse más que lo hace usualmente.

edicinas:

stas recetas de medicina se las dieron para que se las tome en casa:

Methergine 0.2 mg para tomar cada 4 horas. Esto le ayudará a su utero a retornar a su tamaño normal.

Vibramycin 250 mg para tomar 2 veces al día. Estos son antibióticos para prevenir infección.

Tylenol con codeína para el dolor. Puede tomar una o dos pastillas cada 4 horas cuando lo necesita.

] ______________________________

____

] Llame por teléfono para hacer una cita en la Clínica de Ginecología (Clínica de Mujeres) en __________ semanas.

] Vaya con su doctor particular o vaya a la clínica de salud en __________ semanas.

LAME POR TELEFONO O REGRESE A LA SALA DE EMERGENCIA SI LE PASA O SIGUIENTE

. Si le aumenta el flujo de sangre o si su sangre se vuelve de color muy rojo.
. Si pasa coágulos muy grandes de sangre o tejido de la vagina.
. Si tiene fiebre más alta que 100 grados F o 38 grados C.
. Si tiene aumento de dolor o cólicos.
. Si tiene desechos de la vagina de mal olor.

ranslated from English to Spanish by Pauline Manzanares, Denver General Hospital Spanish nterpreter.

ECTOPIC PREGNANCY (POSSIBLE)

GENERAL INFORMATION

You were seen and evaluated in the emergency department for abdominal pain on t date ________________________. One of the possibilities considered in our evaluati was an ectopic pregnancy (a pregnancy in one of your tubes or elsewhere in the dominal cavity).

INSTRUCTIONS

We have done the tests and examinations available to us and feel it is appropriate you to go home.

CALL OR RETURN TO THE EMERGENCY DEPARTMENT

1. If there is any abnormal vaginal bleeding.
2. If the abdominal pain increases.
3. If you have pain in either shoulder.
4. If you have fainting.

RE: ECTOPIC PREGNANCY (POSSIBLE)

1BARAZO ECTOPICO (POSIBLE)

FORMACION GENERAL

usted la examinaron y la evaluaron en la Sala de Emergencia para dolor de estómago la fecha ______________________. Una de las posibilidades que se consideró en estra evaluación fue un embarazo ectópico (un embarazo en uno de sus tubos o en ro lugar en la cavidad del abdomen).

STRUCCIONES

emos hecho todas las pruebas y exámenes que podemos hacer y pensamos que sería ejor que usted regrese a su casa.

AME POR TELEFONO O REGRESE A LA SALA DE EMERGENCIA SI LE PASA) SIGUIENTE

Si sangra anormal de la vagina.
Si el dolor de su estómago aumenta.
Si tiene dolor en cualquier hombro.
Si se desmaya.

---

anslated from English to Spanish by Pauline Manzanares, Denver General Hospital Spanish terpreter.

HEAD INJURY

GENERAL INFORMATION

You have an injury involving your head. This may involve a small bruise or it may b more serious. At this time, we have found no evidence of serious brain or skull injur However, another person needs to observe you for the next 24 hours at home. Shoul your condition worsen, this person needs to call or return you to the emergency de partment.

After a head injury, it is normal for you:

- to have a headache.
- to have mild nausea and one or two episodes of vomiting.
- to be mildly dizzy or drowsy.

INSTRUCTIONS

1. You may take aspirin or Tylenol every 4 hours for pain. DO NOT take any stronge medications.
2. Do not drink any alcoholic beverages for 24 hours.
3. Have someone wake you up every ________ hours for 24 hours and check you fo complications (see below).

SPECIFIC INSTRUCTIONS FOR CHILDREN

1. Awaken child every 2 hours for 24 hours; make sure child can walk and talk.
2. DO NOT give child any pain medications. If headache is severe, bring the child bac to the emergency department.

CALL OR RETURN TO THE EMERGENCY DEPARTMENT

1. If you exhibit increased sleepiness or confusion (inability to wake up completely).
2. If you have an increased headache.
3. If you vomit more than three times.
4. If you have changes in behavior.
5. If you have slurred speech.
6. If you have weakness in arms or legs.
7. If you are stumbling.
8. If you have seizures (convulsions).
9. If you develop unequal pupils (the dark areas in the center of the eye are not th same size).
10. If you have blurred vision.

RE: HEAD INJURY

RIDA DE LA CABEZA

'ORMACION GENERAL

ed tiene una herida en su cabeza. Esto puede ser un moretón pequeño o puede ser ; grave. Ahora no hemos encontrado ninguna herida grave del cerebro o del cráneo. embargo, otra persona tiene que observarlo por las próximas 24 horas en su casa. Si :ondición empeora, esta persona tiene que llamar o traerlo a la Sala de Emergencia.

spués de una herida de la cabeza, es normal para usted:
ue tenga dolor de cabeza.
ue tenga poca náusea o que vomite una o dos veces.
ue esté un poco mareado o soñoliento.

STRUCCIONES

Puede tomar aspirina o Tylenol para el dolor cada 4 horas. NO TOME otra medicina más fuerte.
No beba ninguna bebida alcohólica por 24 horas.
Tenga alguién que lo despierte cada ________ horas por 24 horas y que le revise las complicaciones escritas abajo.

STRUCCIONES ESPECIFICAS PARA NIÑOS

Despierte el niño cada 2 horas por 24 horas; esté seguro que el niño puede caminar y hablar.
NO le dé medicina para el dolor al niño. Si él tiene dolor de cabeza muy fuerte, tráigalo otra vez a la Sala de Emergencia.

AME POR TELEFONO O REGRESE A LA SALA DE EMERGENCIA SI LE PASA SIGUIENTE

. Si le aumenta el sueño o confusión (si no puede despertar completamente).
. Si le aumenta los dolores de cabeza.
. Si vomita más de 3 veces.
. Si tiene cambios en la manera de portarse.
. Si pronuncia indistintamente las palabras cuando habla.
. Si tiene debilidad en los brazos o las piernas.
. Si está tropezando.
. Si le da ataques (convulsiones).
. Si tiene desarrollo de las pupilas desiguales (que los áreas en el medio de los ojos no son del mismo tamaño).
. Si se le empaña la vista.

---

nslated from English to Spanish by Pauline Manzanares, Denver General Hospital Spanish erpreter.

LOW BACK PAIN

GENERAL INFORMATION

Low back pain can be caused by several things. The pain may be related to bone, mu cle, ligament, or nerve injury. You may have never had back problems when for vario reasons you began to have pain. You may also be able to pinpoint the exact activity th produced the pain. The pain may stay in your back or it may travel. It will usually be a ache but it can be very sharp and painful. It may take several days for the pain decrease, so be patient. In order to speed healing and reduce the pain, we advise you follow these instructions.

INSTRUCTIONS

Activity:

- Limit your activity to what you can tolerate without pain.
- For the first day or two stay flat in bed, getting up only to go to the bathroom and eat.
- Rest on a firm surface (carpeted floor or firm mattress) with a pillow under the knee or on your side with knees bent. This will help relax your muscles (a piece plywood between your mattress and box springs may help).
- Avoid high-heeled shoes.

Heat:

- Apply heat to your back by using hot soaks, heating pads, warm baths, or whirlpool Use for 30 minutes every 3 to 4 hours.
- Use gentle massage to reduce pain.

Medication:

☐ You have been given this medication: ______________________________

____

____

CALL OR RETURN TO THE EMERGENCY DEPARTMENT

1. If you have numbness or weakness in your legs.
2. If you have shooting pains into buttocks, groin, or legs.
3. If you have problems with urination.
4. If your pain gets worse.

RE: LOW BACK PAIN

OLOR DE ESPALDA

NFORMACION GENERAL

olor de espalda puede ser causado por muchas cosas. El dolor puede ser relacionado on el hueso, músculo, ligamento, o lastimadura de un nervio. Tal vez nunca ha tenido roblemas de la espalda, cuando por razones variadas empieza a tener dolor. Probable-ente, podrá determinar la actividad exacta que produce el dolor. El dolor se podrá uedar en su espalda o tal vez podrá trasladarse a otro lugar. Usualmente, será un mal-star pero también puede ser un dolor muy agudo. Tal vez tomará muchos días para que disminuya el dolor, así que tenga paciencia. Para que sane rápido y reducir el dolor, ecomendamos que siga estas instrucciones.

NSTRUCCIONES

ctividad:

Limite sus actividades a lo que puede tolerar sin dolor.

Por el primer día o dos manténgase de plano en la cama, levantándose sólo para ir al baño y para comer.

Descanse en un lugar firme (como en un piso con alfombra o un colchón duro) con una almohada debajo de sus rodillas, o descanse a su lado con sus rodillas dobladas. Esto ayudará relajar sus músculos (un pedazo de madera terciada entre su colchón y el colchón de muelles puede ayudar).

Evite zapatos de tacón alto.

alor:

Aplíquese calor a su espalda con compresas calientes, almohada eléctrica, baños en agua caliente, o un remolino. Use cualquiera de estas cosas por 30 minutos cada 3 a 4 horas.

Use un masaje suave para reducir el dolor.

edicina:

☐ Le han dado estas medicinas: ______________________________

____

____

LAME POR TELEFONO O REGRESE A LA SALA DE EMERGENCIA SI LE PASA O SIGUIENTE

1. Si tiene entumecimiento o debilidad en sus piernas.
2. Si siente punzadas en las sentaduras, ingle o piernas.
3. Si tiene problemas al orinar.
4. Si su dolor se empeora.

ranslated from English to Spanish by Pauline Manzanares, Denver General Hospital Spanish nterpreter.

MISCARRIAGE, THREATENED

GENERAL INFORMATION

A small amount of bleeding from the vagina is common in early pregnancy. Sometime this bleeding is normal but sometimes it is a sign that your body is trying to end th pregnancy. This is called a threatened abortion or miscarriage. Your examination show that you are still pregnant.

INSTRUCTIONS

1. Rest in bed until the bleeding stops. You may get up to use the bathroom.
2. Do not put anything into your vagina for 1 week after the bleeding has stopped.
3. Do not have intercourse, use tampons, or douche until your next GYN appointment.
4. If your bleeding stops after 24 hours, participate in only moderate activity for 2 weeks and do not have intercourse for 2 weeks.
5. If you have no further problems, keep your regular GYN appointment (or privat doctor). If you are not being followed by a doctor for your pregnancy, you mus make an appointment to be seen within 2 weeks in the GYN clinic.

CALL OR RETURN TO THE EMERGENCY DEPARTMENT

1. If you experience increased bleeding.
2. If you pass large clots or material that looks like tissue (save anything you pass from your vagina to bring back to the emergency department).
3. If you have cramping in your stomach or back.

RE: MISCARRIAGE, THREATENED

MENAZO DE ABORTO ESPONTANEO

FORMACION GENERAL

poco de sangre le sale de la vagina eso es común durante el principio del embarazo. gunas veces esta sangre es normal pero algunas veces es una señal que su cuerpo está atando de terminar el embarazo. Esto se llama amenazo de aborto espontáneo. Su aminación indica que usted todavía está embarazada.

STRUCCIONES

Descanse en cama hasta que deje de sangrar. Puede levantarse de la cama para ir al baño.

No se meta nada en la vagina por 1 semana después de que pare de sangrar.

No tenga relaciones sexuales, no use tampones, y no se ponga lavados hasta después de su próxima cita con el ginecólogo.

Si deja de sangrar después de 24 horas, solamente haga actividades moderadas por 2 semanas y no tenga relaciones sexuales por 2 semanas.

Si no tiene más problemas, cumpla con su cita con el ginecólogo (o con su doctor particular). Si un doctor no la está revisando regularmente por su embarazo, debe de hacer una cita para que le revisen en 2 semanas aquí en la Clínica de Ginecología (Clínica de Mujeres).

LAME POR TELEFONO O REGRESE A LA SALA DE EMERGENCIA SI LE PASA O SIGUIENTE

Si tiene aumento de sangre.

Si pasa coágulos grandes o material que se parece a tejido (guarde todo lo que pasa por la vagina para traerlo a la Sala de Emergencia).

Si tiene calambres en su estómago o su espalda.

---

anslated from English to Spanish by Pauline Manzanares, Denver General Hospital Spanish terpreter.

NOSEBLEEDS

GENERAL INFORMATION

Nosebleeds are often caused by injuring a blood vessel in the nose with Q-Tips, finge tips, by vigorous nose blowing, or by injury to the nose. They can also be caused b dryness, high blood pressure, infections, allergies, and blood diseases.

INSTRUCTIONS

1. Do not pick your nose or insert anything into it. Do not blow your nose with force
2. Avoid stooping or heavy lifting for 24 hours.
3. If you sneeze, do so through your mouth.
4. Put a little Vaseline inside your nose to help relieve dryness and irritation. This wi also soften the crusts that form after a nosebleed. Do this for 7 days.
5. Increase the moisture in your home with a humidifier, a pan of water on the radiato or a vaporizer.
6. Do not take aspirin for 5 days. This may start the bleeding again.

If the bleeding starts again:

1. Sit up with your head slightly forward. Pinch the entire soft part of the nose close for 10 minutes. Breath through your mouth and spit out blood through your mouth.

☐ Packing has been left in your nose:

- DO NOT pull it out. If part of the packing starts to come out, either cut it off o tuck it back in.
- Apply cold compresses over the nose to help relieve the pressure of the packing.
- Call to make an appointment in the ear, nose, and throat (ENT) clinic in ______ days to have your packing removed.

CALL OR RETURN TO THE EMERGENCY DEPARTMENT

1. If you have bleeding that you are unable to stop.
2. If there is bleeding through the pack or into the back of the throat.
3. If there is pus-like drainage from the nose.
4. If you have increasing pain in the nose.
5. If you have swelling of the nose that makes breathing difficult.
6. If you continue to have frequent nosebleeds.

RE: NOSEBLEEDS

:MORRAGIAS NASALES

FORMACION GENERAL

morragias nasales con frecuencia son causadas por una lastimadura del vaso guíneo de la nariz con Q-tips (palitos con algodón), puntas de los dedos o por iarse las narices fuertemente, o por una lastimadura de la nariz. También se pueden ısar por sequedad, presión alta, infecciones, alergias, y enfermedades de la sangre.

STRUCCIONES

No debe de picarse la nariz o meterse algo a dentro. No debe de sonarse la nariz con mucha fuerza.

Evite agacharse o levantar cosas pesadas por 24 horas.

Si destornuda, hágalo por la boca.

Póngase un poco de Vaselina adentro de la nariz para que le ayuda a aliviar la sequedad e irritación. Esto también le ablandará la costra que se forma después de una hemorragia nasal. Hago esto por 7 días.

Aumente la humedad en su casa con un humedecedor, una cacerola de agua sobre un radiador (aparato de calefacción), o una vaporizadora.

No tome aspirina por 5 días. Eso puede causar que comience a sangrar otra vez.

comienza sangrar otra vez:

Siéntese con su cabeza poco adelantada. Apriete y mantenga cerrada toda la parte blanda de su nariz por 10 minutos. Respire por su boca y escupa la sangre por su boca.

Han dejado las compresas adentro de su nariz:

- NO se las saque. Si parte de las compresas comienzan a salir, córtelas o póngalas dentro de la nariz otra vez.
- Póngase compresas frías sobre la nariz para que le ayude a aliviar la presión de las compresas adentro de la nariz.
- Llame por teléfono para hacer una cita en la Clínica de Ojos, Nariz, y Garganta (ENT Clinic) en ________ días para que le quiten las compresas.

LAME POR TELEFONO O REGRESE A LA SALA DE EMERGENCIA SI LE PASA O SIGUIENTE

Si tiene mucho flujo de sangre que no puede parar.

Si tiene flujo de sangre por las compresas que tiene adentro de la nariz o si tiene flujo de sangre hacia detrás de la garganta.

Si tiene drenaje como pus de la nariz.

. Si tiene aumento de dolor de la nariz.

. Si tiene hinchazón de la nariz que hace la respiración difícil.

. Si usted continúa con hemorragias nasales frecuentemente.

ranslated from English to Spanish by Pauline Manzanares, Denver General Hospital Spanish nterpreter.

GONORRHEA/PELVIC INFLAMMATORY DISEASE (PID)

GENERAL INFORMATION

You have an infection in your female organs (uterus or ovaries and fallopian tubes). Th infection can be a persistent problem. Be sure to follow your treatment as directed the infection will get worse.

Symptoms:

- Lower abdominal pain
- Occasional fever and chills.
- Vaginal discharge may be present.

INSTRUCTIONS

1. Drink 6 to 8 full glasses of liquid (8 ounces) every day.
2. Take medications as instructed by your doctor. Make sure you take all the antibiotic given to you, even if you feel better. Your symptoms should begin to get better in 2 to 36 hours.
3. No sexual intercourse for 2 weeks.
4. Please make and keep an appointment for follow-up in the GYN clinic or with you private physician.
5. Ask sexual contacts to call the VD clinic so they can be checked for infection an treated.

CALL OR RETURN TO THE EMERGENCY DEPARTMENT

1. If you have increased pain or vaginal bleeding.
2. If your temperature goes up to 101 degrees F or 38 degrees C.
3. If you have increased vaginal discharge.
4. If you develop a rash or questionable reaction from medication.

RE: GONORRHEA/PELVIC INFLAMMATORY DISEASE (PID)

NORREA/ENFERMEDAD DE INFLAMACION DE LA PELVIS

ORMACION GENERAL

ed tiene una infección en sus órganos femeninos (útero u ovarios y trompas de pio). Esto puede ser un problema persistente. Esté segura de seguir el tratamiento omendado o la infección va a empeorar.

tomas:

olor abdominal más bajo.
iebre y escalofríos ocasionales.
uede tener desecho vaginal.

TRUCCIONES

Tome 6 a 8 vasos llenos de líquidos (8 onzas) cada día.
Tome las medicinas como ha prescrito su doctor. Esté segura que tome todos los antibióticos que le han dado, aunque se sienta mejor. Sus síntomas deben mejorar en 24 a 36 horas.
No tenga relaciones sexuales por 2 semanas.
Por favor haga y cumpla con citas de tratamiento complementario en la Clínica de Ginecología o con su doctor particular.
Pida a su compañero con quien ha tenido relaciones sexuales que llame a la Clínica de Enfermedad Venérea.

AME POR TELEFONO O REGRESE A LA SALA DE EMERGENCIA SI LE PASA SIGUIENTE

Si le ha aumentado el dolor o si sangra de la vagina.
Si su temperatura le sube a 101 grados F o 38 grados C.
Si le aumenta el desecho vaginal.
Si le desarrolla ronchas, o si tiene una reacción dudosa por la medicina.

---

nslated from English to Spanish by Pauline Manzanares, Denver General Hospital Spanish erpreter.

SPRAINS AND FRACTURES

GENERAL INFORMATION

A sprain is an injury to the tissues that hold the joints together. Sprains produce varyi degrees of stretching or tearing of a ligament. A fracture is a break in the bone. Bo sprains and fractures cause pain and swelling. They must be protected and immobiliz until they heal. Some of these injuries may require a cast or Ace wrap until they he properly. It is recommended you care for your injury in the following manner:

INSTRUCTIONS

Immobilization:

- ☐ A cast has been applied. Follow instructions on your follow-up sheet.
- ☐ Wear the splint or Ace wrap provided. This rests the injured part and allows it heal. If you wear an Ace wrap, adjust it for comfort. Make sure it is tight enough f you to feel support but not so tight that you feel numbness or tingling. Remove ar reapply the Ace wrap once a day.

Elevation:

Elevate the injured part to reduce swelling. With pillows place the injured part abo the level of the heart. Elevation is most important in the first 24 hours.

Cold:

Cold helps reduce further pain and swelling. Apply cold packs for 15 to 30 minut every 1 to 2 hours for the first 48 hours. Place ice in a plastic or rubber bag and cover with a dry cloth to protect the skin or cast.

Heat:

Do not apply heat for the first 48 hours after your injury. If you use heat too early, it w increase the pain and swelling. After 48 hours, use warm packs or warm soaks for 3 minutes only, 2 to 4 hours daily. The heat will help reduce stiffness and soreness.

Activity:

Do not bear weight on the injured part as long as it is painful. Use crutches or a cane a you were instructed. Gradually bear weight as the pain decreases. If you have a walkin cast, do not walk on it for 24 hours.

CALL OR RETURN TO THE EMERGENCY DEPARTMENT

1. If the pain and symptoms persist for 8 to 10 days.
2. If there is increased swelling.
3. If there is increased pain.
4. If there is numbness.
5. If there is coldness of skin.
6. If you have a change of skin or nail color to blue.

RE: SPRAINS AND FRACTURES

)RCEDURAS Y FRACTURAS

FORMACION GENERAL

a torcedura es una herida de los tejidos que mantienen las coyunturas juntas. Torceras producen grados variados de estiraje o rotura de un ligamento. Una fractura es a quebradura del hueso. Ambos torceduras y fracturas causan dolor e hinchazón. enen que ser protejidos e inmovilizados hasta que sanen. Algunos de estas heridas eden requerir un yeso o una banda elástica (Ace wrap) hasta que sanen. Está recoendado que usted cuide su herida en la manera siguiente:

'STRUCCIONES

movilización:

Le han puesto un yeso. Siga las instrucciones en la página que le han dado para tratamiento complementario.

Use la tablilla o banda elástica que le han dado. Esto descansará la parte herida y la deja que sane. Si usa una banda elástica, ajústela para mantenerla cómoda. Esté seguro que la banda elástica está suficientemente apretada para que le dé soporte pero no tan apretada que sienta entumecimiento u hormigueo. Una vez al día quítese la banda elástica y póngasela otra vez.

evación:

ra reducir la hinchazón pónga la parte herida más alta que el nivel del corazón usando mohadas. Esto es muy importante hacer en las primeras 24 horas.

ío:

ío ayuda reducir más dolor e hinchazón. Póngase compresas frías por 15 a 30 minutos da una o dos horas por las primeras 48 horas. Pónga hielo en una bolsa de plástico o goma y cúbralo con una tela seca para proteger la piel o el yeso.

alor:

o se aplique calor por las primeras 48 horas después que se lastimó. Si usa el calor muy onto, aumentará el dolor y la hinchazón. Después de 48 horas, use compresas lientes o remojos calientes por sólo 30 minutos cada 2 a 4 horas diarias. Esto ayudará reducir la tiesura y la parte adolorida.

ctividad:

o pónga peso en la parte herida mientras le duele. Use muletas o un bastón como le an dicho. Gradualmente ponga peso en la parte herida tal como se disminuya el dolor. está usando un yeso de caminar, no camine en él por 24 horas.

LAME POR TELEFONO O REGRESE A LA SALA DE EMERGENCIA SI LE PASA O SIGUIENTE

. Si el dolor y síntomas persisten por 8 a 10 días.
. Si le aumenta la hinchazón.
. Si le aumenta el dolor.
. Si tiene entumecimiento.
. Si tiene la piel fría.
. Si la piel o las uñas se cambian a color azul.

---

ranslated from English to Spanish by Pauline Manzanares, Denver General Hospital Spanish iterpreter.

URINARY TRACT INFECTIONS

GENERAL INFORMATION

The most common site of the urinary infection known as cystitis is the bladder.

Symptoms:

1. Need to urinate more often (frequency).
2. Need to urinate right away and can't hold it (urgency).
3. Burning with urination (dysuria).
4. Occasionally blood in the urine.

Pyelonephritis is an infection involving the kidneys.

Symptoms:

1. Frequency, urgency, dysuria.
2. Flank (side) pain.
3. Fever and chills.
4. Occasionally nausea and vomiting.

INSTRUCTIONS

1. You have been given an antibiotic to treat the infection. Take it according to the physician's instructions.
2. A urine sample has been sent to the lab. You will be notified if further treatment is needed.
3. Drink 6 to 8 glasses of water a day.
4. Avoid long periods between urination. Try to empty your bladder every 3 hours.
5. After bowel movements, wipe from front to back to avoid contaminating the urethral opening.
6. Return to the emergency department or walk-in clinic for follow-up urine cultures if requested by physician.

CALL OR RETURN TO THE EMERGENCY DEPARTMENT OR WALK-IN CLINIC

1. If you cannot keep your medicines down because of vomiting.
2. If your medicines cause allergic reactions such as skin rash, hives, itching, wheezing.
3. If your temperature remains elevated after 48 hours of treatment.

RE: URINARY TRACT INFECTIONS

IFECCIONES DE VIAS URINARIAS

IFORMACION GENERAL

vejiga es el sitio más común de la infección urinaria conocida como cistitis.

ıtomas:

Se ha aumentado la frecuencia de orinar.
Le urge orinar más frecuentemente y no lo puede detener (urgencia).
Le arde cuando orina (disuria).
De vez en cuando hay sangre en la orina.

elonefritis es una infección envolviendo los riñones.

ntomas:

Frecuencia, urgencia, disuria.
Dolor de flanco (lado).
Fiebre y escalofríos.
De vez en cuando tiene náusea y vómitos.

ISTRUCCIONES

Le han dado un antibiótico para curar la infección. Tómela según las instrucciones de su doctor.
Han mandado una muestra de orina al laboratorio. Le avisarán si es necesario darle tratamiento adicional.
Tome 6 a 8 vasos de agua diario.
Evite períodos largos entre urinación. Trate de vaciar su vejiga cada 3 horas.
Después de hacer del baño (defecar) límpiese las partes de adelante hacia atrás para evitar contaminar la apertura de la uretra.
Regrese a la Clínica de Emergencia (walk-in clinic) para dar otras muestras de orina en caso que su doctor lo requiere.

LAME POR TELEFONO O REGRESE A LA SALA DE EMERGENCIA WALK-IN CLINIC) SI LE PASA LO SIGUIENTE

. No puede mantener las medicinas en su cuerpo y las está vomitando.
. Su medicina causa reacción de alergia, como salpullido, ronchas, picazón, resuello difícil y ronco.
. Su temperatura todavía está alta después de 48 horas de tratamiento.

---

ranslated from English to Spanish by Pauline Manzanares, Denver General Hospital Spanish iterpreter.

VOMITING AND DIARRHEA

GENERAL INFORMATION

Vomiting and diarrhea are usually caused by a viral infection of the intestines. We hav done the tests and examinations that were indicated and feel that your illness can b treated at home.

The only real danger in having vomiting or diarrhea is dehydration. It is importa for you to take fluids in such a way that you will be able to keep them down. Th following diet will be helpful to you. It is suggested you follow it for 24 to 48 hour

INSTRUCTIONS

1. Diet: Clear tea, decaffeinated coffee, carbonated beverages, Gatorade, Jell-O, app juice, cranberry juice (avoid orange, tomato, grapefruit juice), clear broth, and har candy.
2. If the above diet is tolerated well, progress to dry toast (no jelly or butter), bouillo or other clear soups. Avoid any dairy products for 24 hours after diarrhea ha stopped.
3. You may resume a normal diet at the end of 48 hours. However, avoid spicy food fried foods, and raw fruits for a few more days.
4. Wash hands thoroughly after using the restroom.

CALL OR RETURN TO THE EMERGENCY DEPARTMENT

1. If your stomach pain becomes more severe than the occasional cramps.
2. If you vomit blood or "coffee-ground" drainage.
3. If you have bloody diarrhea.
4. If you experience frequent and severe vomiting and diarrhea.
5. If you have these signs of dehydration:
   - decreased urination or dark urine
   - weakness
   - dizziness when standing

RE: VOMITING AND DIARRHEA

OMITOS Y DIARREA

NFORMACION GENERAL

ómitos y diarrea usualmente están causados por una infección de virus de los intesti-os. Hemos hecho todas las pruebas y examinaciones necesarias y pensamos que esto se uede curar en casa.

El único peligro en tener vómitos y diarrea es deshidratación. Es importante que sted tome líquidos de una manera que pueda mantenerlos en el cuerpo. La siguiente ieta le ayudará. Está recomendado que la siga por 24 a 48 horas.

NSTRUCCIONES

. Dieta: Té claro, café sin cafeína, bebidas carbonatadas, Gatorade (soda), gelatina, jugo de manzana, jugo de arándano (evite jugos de naranja, tomate, y toronja), caldo claro, y dulces duros.
. Si la dieta de arriba se puede tolerar bien, entonces puede comer pan tostado seco (no le ponga jalea o mantequilla), caldo, u otras sopas claras. Evite cualquier producto lechero por 24 horas después que ha parado la diarrea.
. Puede reasumir una dieta normal después de 48 horas. Sin embargo, evite comidas picantes, comidas fritas, y frutas crudas por unos cuantos días más.
. Lávase las manos bien después de ir al baño.

LAME POR TELEFONO O REGRESE A LA SALA DE EMERGENCIA SI LE PASA O SIGUIENTE

. Si el dolor de su estómago se pone más severo de los calambres ocasionales.
. Si vomita sangre o si tiene drenaje que se parece a borras del café.
. Si tiene diarrea sangrienta.
. Si tiene vómitos o diarrea frecuentemente o graves.
. Si tiene estas señales de deshidratación:
  - urinación disminuída u orina obscura
  - debilidad
  - mareos cuando se para

---

ranslated from English to Spanish by Pauline Manzanares, Denver General Hospital Spanish nterpreter.

WOUND AND LACERATION CARE

GENERAL INFORMATION

When the body tissues have been damaged by a cut, burn, or abrasion, they must protected and watched carefully for infection. Despite the best of care, there is alway chance that such wounds may be infected by bacteria or other germs.

INSTRUCTIONS

1. *Elevate the injured area:* propping the injured area up on pillows will reduce sw ing and therefore pain.
2. *Bandage care:* keep your dressing clean and dry and follow any specific instructic given by your physician.
3. *Stitches:* return to the emergency department in ________ days to have the stitch removed. For facial stitches, cleanse with half-strength hydrogen peroxide and wa twice a day. All other stitches should be kept clean and dry for 24 hours. Follow other specific instructions given by doctor:

   ____

   ____
4. *Wound re-check:* return for wound check in ________ days.
5. *Medicine:* if you have been given antibiotics, take ALL the medicine prescribed. you have been given pain medicines, take them as prescribed; otherwise, take aspi or Tylenol every 4 hours.
6. *Infection:* be alert for signs of infection as listed below.

CALL OR RETURN TO THE EMERGENCY DEPARTMENT

1. If there is redness, swelling, tenderness.
2. If there is pus draining from the wound.
3. If you have chills, fever.
4. If there are tender lumps in your groin or armpit.
5. If there are red streaks going up your arm or leg.

RE: WOUND AND LACERATION CARE

CUIDADO DE HERIDA Y LACERACION

INFORMACION GENERAL

Cuando los tejidos del cuerpo han sido dañados de una cortada, quemadura, o abrasión, tienen que ser protegidos y observados cuidadosamente para infección. A pesar del mejor cuidado, siempre hay la posibilidad de que tales heridas se pueden infectar por bacterias u otros microbios.

INSTRUCCIONES

1. *Levante el área herida:* Mantenga el área herida hacia arriba en el aire con almohadas. Reducirá la hinchazón y debido a eso, el dolor.
2. *Cuidado del vendaje:* Mantenga su vendaje limpio y seco y siga exactamente las instrucciones especiales que le ha dado su doctor.
3. *Puntadas:* Regrese a la Sala de Emergencia en ________ días para que le quiten las puntadas. Para puntadas en la cara, límpiese la cara con la mitad de agua oxigenada y la mitad de agua, dos veces al día. Mantenga otras puntadas limpias y secas por 24 horas. Siga todas las demás instrucciones especiales que le ha dado su doctor:
____
____
4. *Chequeo de herida:* Regrese por un chequeo de su herida en ________ días.
5. *Medicina:* Si le han dado antibióticos, tome TODA la medicina que le han recetado. Si le han dado medicina para dolor, tómela como su doctor la recetó; si no le han dado medicina para dolor, tome aspirina o Tylenol cada 4 horas.
6. *Infección:* Esté alerto por las señales de infección que se indican abajo.

LLAME POR TELEFONO O REGRESE A LA SALA DE EMERGENCIA SI LE PASA LO SIGUIENTE

1. Si tiene enrojecimiento, hinchazón, o dolencia.
2. Si le sale pus de la herida.
3. Si tiene fiebre o escalofríos.
4. Si tiene nudos (bolitas) en la ingle o debajo del brazo que le duelan.
5. Si tiene rayas rojas en el brazo o en la pierna.

Translated from English to Spanish by Pauline Manzanares, Denver General Hospital Spanish Interpreter.

DIARRHEA (CHILD)

GENERAL INFORMATION

Diarrhea (loose watery bowel movement) is a common problem of growing childre Once in a while diarrhea may be caused by serious illness but usually it is only a min problem. It is usually caused by a viral infection of the intestines and can last sever days to a week. However, if your child loses too much water, he or she becomes d hydrated (dried out) and can get very sick. This can usually be prevented by increasi the amount of fluids your child takes.

INSTRUCTIONS

Treatment (for the infant who is not toilet-trained):

1. Have the baby take just clear fluids (ones you can see through) for the first 24 hou Examples of clear fluids are apple juice, ice popsicles, tea, Jell-O (use twice as muc water as usual), soda pop (with the bubbles shaken out), weak broth, or Gatorade
2. Use combinations of the above liquids throughout the day. Give the liquids in sma amounts quite often. If the diarrhea improves within 24 hours, go next to ha strength formula or half-strength skim milk. If the baby is old enough to eat sc foods, you can go to the following: applesauce, bananas, simple unsalted cracker carrot juice, or rice cereal.
3. If the baby has no more diarrhea, gradually go back to full-strength milk or formu and the usual diet for age by day 3 or 4. If runny bowels reoccur, start over aga with clear fluids.*

CALL THE EMERGENCY DEPARTMENT PHONE NUMBER

1. If the child suddenly develops a high fever.
2. If stomach pain becomes severe (lasts over 2 hours).
3. If there is any blood, pus, or mucus in the diarrhea.
4. If the diarrhea becomes more frequent or more severe.
5. If there is no improvement after 24 hours.
6. If there are signs of dehydration—such as decrease in urine or wet diapers, weigh loss, dry tongue or mouth, no tears when the child cries, less activity than usua sunken eyes.

If you have any questions or concerns call the Pediatric Clinic.
AFTER 11:00 PM call the emergency department.

*Do not use stool binders for children unless you are directed to do so by your doctor.

VER (CHILD)

NERAL INFORMATION

ever is a rise in body temperature above normal. If your child looks flushed, is rest-s, and has a hot skin, he or she may have a fever. Take your child's temperature. If the tal temperature is above 103 degrees F, the temperature must be lowered to normal. e way to help the fever come down is to give the child a sponge bath in a tub.

STRUCTIONS

rections for sponge bath:

Fill the tub with 2 inches of water that is warm to your wrist.
Wet and partially wring out a washcloth.
Sponge the child's body with the washcloth (use long, soothing strokes over face, neck, arms, chest, back, and legs).
Sponge for 20 minutes.
Remove child from tub and cover him or her with a light blanket.
Wait 30 minutes and take the child's temperature.
If the temperature is still high, repeat the bath until the temperature is 101 degrees F measured rectally.
If the child starts to shiver, stop sponging and remove the child from the tub. When shivering stops, warm the water and put the child back in the tub.

eventive care:

To help keep the temperature normal, give clear liquids. The child can drink as much water and juice as he or she will take.
Your child may have ________________ every ________ hours. Give this as directed by the doctor. DO NOT give your child aspirin unless directed to by the physician.

LL THE EMERGENCY DEPARTMENT PHONE NUMBER

If your child's fever goes above 104 degrees F or 41 degrees C.
If the fever remains above 103 degrees F after the above treatment.
If the fever lasts for 72 hours.
If your child is less than 3 months old.
If your child has anything resembling a convulsion.
If he or she has a stiff neck, confusion, or delirium ("out of his head").
If he or she has difficulty breathing.
If he or she has purple spots on the skin.
If he or she has burning with urination or is urinating more frequently.

you have any questions or concerns call the Pediatric Clinic.
TER 11:00 PM call the emergency department.

HEAD INJURY (CHILD)

GENERAL INFORMATION

Your child has had a head injury and is now ready to go home. There are a few thi you need to do and watch for. Listed below are signs of head injury. If you see an these signs, call the emergency department or come in.

INSTRUCTIONS

Signs of head injury:

1. Changes in your child's behavior, such as extreme irritability.
2. Nausea (upset stomach).
3. Vomiting (throwing up).
4. Headache or stiff neck.
5. Bleeding from ears or nose.
6. Increased sleepiness, difficult to wake up.
7. Temperature more than 101 degrees F or 38 degrees C.
8. Convulsions (seizures).
9. Staggering or swaying while walking.
10. Weakness on one side of the body.
11. Eye changes (crossed eyes, droopy eyelids, trouble seeing, blurry vision, or see double).
12. Loss of consciousness (does not awaken when you speak or touch him or her
13. If your child does not "look right" to you.

Your child should avoid rough activity until after his or her follow-up visit with doctor. Call the emergency department if you have any questions.

)MITING (CHILD)

ENERAL INFORMATION

ost vomiting is caused by a viral infection of the intestinal tract or your child eating mething that has not agreed with him or her. The following dietary changes usually eed recovery.

STRUCTIONS

eatment:

u should give small amounts of clear liquids often (1 to 2 ounces every 20 minutes r a few hours). You can give soda pop with the fizz shaken out (Coke, Seven-Up), ple juice, sweetened weak tea, popsicles, Gatorade, water, or 1 or 2 tablespoons of ney or Karo syrup in a small amount of cool water. If your child takes these fluids ell, allow him or her to increase the amount. If the child vomits, wait 1 hour before fering more liquids. If your child wants solid foods and you think he or she can hold em down, try small amounts of soda crackers, graham crackers, vanilla wafers, or asted bread. After 8 hours with no vomiting, your child can return to a normal diet.

ALL THE EMERGENCY DEPARTMENT PHONE NUMBER

- If your child vomits blood or material that looks like coffee grounds.
- If vomiting becomes more severe (continues for more than 12 hours).
- If your child is difficult to awaken or acts confused.
- If your child has constant abdominal pain (stomachache).
- If your child looks dehydrated (dried out). Signs of dehydration are decrease in urine, weight loss, dry tongue or mouth, no tears when he or she cries, less activity than usual, sunken eyes.

you have any questions or concerns call the Pediatric Clinic.

FTER 11:00 PM call the emergency department.

APPENDIX F

LIST OF APPROVED NURSING DIAGNOSES*

Activity intolerance
Activity intolerance, potential
Airway clearance, ineffective
Anxiety
Bowel elimination, alteration in: constipation
Bowel elimination, alteration in: diarrhea
Bowel elimination, alteration in: incontinence
Breathing pattern, ineffective
Cardiac output, alteration in: decreased
Comfort, alteration in: pain
Communication, impaired: verbal
Coping, family: potential for growth
Coping, ineffective family: compromised
Coping, ineffective individual
Diversional activity, deficit
Family process, alteration in
Fear
Fluid volume, alteration in: excess
Fluid volume deficit, actual
Fluid volume deficit, potential
Gas exchange, impaired
Grieving, anticipatory
Grieving, dysfunctional
Health maintenance, alteration in
Home maintenance management, impaired
Injury, potential for: (poisoning, potential for; suffocation, potential for; trauma, pote tial for)
Knowledge deficit (specify)
Mobility, impaired physical

*Kim, M.J., McFarland, G., and McLane, A.M.: Classification of nursing diagnoses: proceedings fifth national conference, St. Louis, 1984, C.V. Mosby Co., pp. 470-471. (The nursing diagnose have been accepted for clinical testing by NANDA.)

ɒncompliance (specify)
ıtrition, alteration in: less than body requirements
ıtrition, alteration in: more than body requirements
ıtrition, alteration in: potential for more than body requirements
ʻal mucous membranes, alteration in
renting, alteration in: actual or potential
ɒwerlessness
ıpe trauma syndrome
lf-care deficit: feeding, bathing/hygiene, dressing/grooming, toileting
lf-concept, disturbance in: body image, self-esteem, role performance, personal identity
nsory-perceptual alteration: visual, auditory, kinesthetic, gustatory, tactile, olfactory
xual dysfunction
:in dysfunction
:in integrity, impairment of: actual
:in integrity, impairment of: potential
eep pattern disturbance
ɔcial isolation
ɔiritual distress (distress of the human spirit)
hought processes, alteration in
issue perfusion, alteration in: cerebral, cardiopulmonary, renal, gastrointestinal, peripheral
rinary elimination, alteration in patterns
iolence, potential for: self-directed or directed at others

BIBLIOGRAPHY

American Heart Association: Algorithms for cardiac dysrhythmias: advanced life support, 1981, The American Heart Association.

American Heart Association: Standards and guidelines for cardiopulmonary resuscitation (CPR) and emergency cardiac care (ECC), JAMA **244:**453, 1980.

Anthony, C.P., and Thibodeau, G.: Textbook of anatomy & physiology, ed. 11, St. Louis, 1983, The C.V. Mosby Co.

Barkin, R.M., and Rosen, P.: Emergency pediatrics, St. Louis, 1984, The C.V. Mosby Co.

Bayer, M.J., and Rumack, B.H., editors: Poisonings and overdose, Top. Emerg. Med. **1**(3), 1979.

Budassi, S.A., and Barber, J.: Emergency nursing: principles and practice, ed. 2, St. Louis, 1985, The C.V. Mosby Co.

Cardiopulmonary resuscitation (CPR) and emergency cardiac care (ECC), JAMA **227** (suppl.):833, 1974.

Chinn, P.L.: Child health maintenance, St. Louis, 1981, The C.V. Mosby Co.

Cosgriff, J., and Anderson, D.: The practice of emergency care, ed. 2, New York, 1984, J.B. Lippincott Co.

Craven, R., and Hedges, J.: Advances in cardiac life support: role of distolic pressure, JEN **10:**204, 1984.

DasGupta, D.: Principles and practices of acute cardiac care, Chicago, 1984, Yearbook Medical Publishers.

Dubovsky, S.L., and Weissberg, M.P.: Clinical psychiatry in primary care, ed. 2, Baltimore, 1982, Williams and Wilkins.

Ehrlich, P.E., editor: Pediatric trauma, Top. Emerg. Med. **4**(3), 1982.

Emergencies, Nurses Reference Library. Springhouse, Penn., 1984, Springhouse Corporation.

Emergency Department Nurses Associati Standards of emergency nursing practice, Louis, 1983, The C.V. Mosby Co.

Emergency Department Nurses Associati core curriculum, Chicago, 1979, Emergen Department Nurses Association.

Emergindex, Denver, Micromedex, Inc. (U dated Quarterly).

Frank, H.A., and Wachtel, T.L., editors: Therm injuries, Top. Emerg. Med. **3**(3), 1981.

Gallagher, E.J., editor: Neurological emerge cies, Top. Emerg. Med. **4**(2), 1982.

Gilman, A.G., Goodman, L.A., and Gilman, The pharmacological basis of therapeuti ed. 6, New York, 1980, Macmillan Publishi Co.

Goldberg, A.H.: Cardio-pulmonary arrest, Engl. J. Med., p. 290, 1974.

Goldhagen, J.L.: Croup: pathogenesis and ma agement, J. Emerg. Med. **1**(1):3, 1983.

Graver, K.: New trends in the management cardiac arrest, Am. Fam. Physician **29**(2 224, 1984.

Grodin, M.A.: Epiglottitis, J. Emerg. Med. **1**(1 13, 1983.

Guzzetta, C., and Dossey, B.: Cardiovascul nursing: bodymind tapestry, St. Louis, 198 The C.V. Mosby Co.

Holland, D.: Cyanide poisoning: an uncommo encounter, JEN **9:**138, 1983.

Holloway, N.: Nursing the critically ill adult, e 2, Menlo Park, Ca., 1984, Addison-Wesley.

Judd, R.L., and Pesyke, M.A., editors: Psycho logical and behavioral emergencies, To Emerg. Med. **4**(4), 1983.

Katz, A.M., and Selwyn, A.: The cardiac a rhythmias, Sunderland, Mass., 1983, Sinaue Association, Inc.

Marx, J.A., and Jordan, R.C., editors: Alcohol related emergencies, Top. Emerg. Med. **6:**2 1984.

cIntyre, K., and Lewis, J., editors: Textbook of advanced life support, Dallas, 1981, American Heart Association.

eislin, H.W., editor: Priorities in multiple trauma, Top. Emerg. Med. **1**:1, 1979.

ethany, N.M., and Snively, M.D.: Nurses' handbook of fluid balance, ed. 4, Philadelphia, 1983, J.B. Lippincott Co.

iller, M.: Pesticide poisoning, JEN **8**:288, 1982.

oore, E., Eiseman, B., VanWay, C.: Critical decisions in trauma, St. Louis, 1984, The C.V. Mosby Co.

user, K., and Spragg, R.: Respiratory emergencies, ed. 2, St. Louis, 1984, The C.V. Mosby Co.

arker, J., editor: Emergency nursing: a guide to comprehensive care, New York, 1983, John Wiley & Sons, Inc.

ierog, J.E., and Pierog, L.J., editors: Pediatric emergencies, Top. Emerg. Med. **3**:1, 1981.

Pierog, L.J., and Deck, K.B., editors: Special aspects of trauma care, Top. Emerg. Med. **6**:1, 1984.

Poisondex, Denver, Micromedex, Inc. (Updated Quarterly).

Price, S.A., and Wilson, L.M.: Physiology clinical concepts of disease processes, New York, 1979, McGraw-Hill Book Co.

Rosen, P., and others: Emergency medicine: concepts and clinical practice, St. Louis, 1983, The C.V. Mosby Co.

Roth, R., Stewart, R., Cannon, G.: Out-of-hospital cardiac arrest: factor associated with survival, Ann. Emerg. Med. **13**(4):237, 1984.

Sahn, S.: Pulmonary emergencies, New York, 1982, Churchill-Livingstone.

Stephens, G.J.: Pathophysiology for health practitioners, New York, 1980, Macmillan Publishing Co.

Sutton, R., Perrins, Citron, P.: Physiological cardiac pacing, PACE **3**:207, 1980.

INDEX

G

H

O

P

R

S

T

Z

CHARLES FREARS COLLEGE OF
NURSING AND MIDWIFERY
LEARNING RESOURCES CENTRE